The
Trauma Informed
Herbalist

A discussion around effectively supporting clients who are struggling with trauma

Elizabeth Guthrie, MPH, RYT500

First paperback edition October 2022

Book cover and illustrations by India J Lott

ISBN 978-1-387-94198-8 (paperback)

www.traumainformedherbalist.com

Dedicated to those in the arena.

Acknowledgements

Thanks to my husband, Josh, for putting up with all of this and still having a sense of humor.

I am extremely appreciative of those who contributed to this work: Dr. Jessica Hoggle for her contribution of content editing the first few chapters and India for the beautiful artwork (and lending an ear when I was overwhelmed).

To all of the other friends, colleagues, family members, and mentors who have encouraged me, I wouldn't be here without my community and I love y'all more than you know.

RIP Elsa, we love you. Your loyalty and protection is what kept me going through the worst of the abuse, and I will always cherish your memory.

Contents

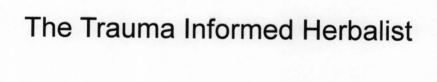

The Trauma Informed Herbalist

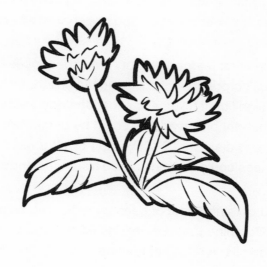

Chapter 1
Introduction

I spent years thinking I needed to toughen up.

The panic attacks, random zapping sensations in my head, and issues with my eyes had gotten overwhelming and I was desperate for answers.

When I first learned that my life experiences qualified as trauma, I was surprised. I had a peaceful childhood and didn't experience significant traumatic situations until I was in my twenties. I thought only war vets could be diagnosed with post traumatic stress disorder (PTSD) and I didn't understand how my experiences could be considered traumatic enough to need help.

I had obtained a lot of secondary trauma as a 911 dispatcher. Combine that with the intimate partner violence I suffered and voilà: A PTSD diagnosis.

I was already using herbs and other natural therapies to help keep physical and emotional balance. Naturally, I began to research how I could apply my knowledge to heal my trauma. I was surprised at what little I found that addressed trauma as its own concern.

Most information I found in natural health circles indicated that relaxation was key. I tried to find ways to relax, but I began to experience heightened trauma symptoms when I would attempt "soothing" activities such as meditation. Many people suggested adaptogens as an option, but the rhodiola I took just made me more hypervigilant. Certain therapies helped, but others made me extremely uncomfortable.

This led to me feeling like something was wrong with me. Why was restorative yoga leaving me so spacey? Why couldn't I drink that herbal tea without feeling on edge?

I soon realized I wasn't alone. As my practice started growing, I saw more clients that didn't benefit from the traditional recommendations. Many of these clients had identifiable trauma that affected their daily lives. I then began to realize how most practitioners understand very little of how trauma rewires the nervous system. It's not as simple as telling your clients to "just relax".

Natural healers need to become trauma-informed

Natural medicine is so powerful, but trauma-informed care is almost non-existent in the field. So few people genuinely understand trauma and how it changes the body and brain's response to stimuli. Many practitioners are inadvertently harming their clients because they are claiming to be trauma-informed without the education necessary to support traumatized clients.

Being trauma-informed is not the same as experiencing trauma. Experiencing trauma only gives you insight into your personal response to a traumatic situation. When I first started studying the trauma response, I was amazed to find that there were so many symptoms attributed to trauma. Many different situations can create trauma responses and everyone will respond uniquely to stressful incidents.

Humans are complex. Our experiences and personalities are as varied as the stars. This means stressors will affect us all differently and I cannot compare my trauma response to yours. Trauma-informed herbalists must acknowledge this and work to create flexibility in our practices that can accommodate this variety.

This book was written to help you brainstorm. Take ideas from my experiences and see how you can apply them to your life and practice. Pay attention to the thought processes I present and consider how that translates into your work.

Trauma-informed work is for everyone

This book was written from a practitioner viewpoint, but many of the principles outlined in these chapters are beneficial for almost anyone. I have found that the more I understand trauma-informed care, the higher my quality of life. Showing compassion to others who are struggling has become easier. Caring for myself by implementing trauma-informed natural modalities has helped me spend more time healing and less time trying to manage my symptoms.

Applying the principles and knowledge of trauma-informed care causes me to hold more empathy for others. Now that I understand how trauma affects us, I have more patience when I am tempted to be frustrated by someone's actions. It has become easier for me to offer compassion and loving kindness toward others.

The herb, aromatherapy, and flower essence chapters hold lists of plants and how I like to use them. Many of these plants have become close allies and have created a sense of safety I could not find elsewhere. I feel privileged to be able to introduce you to these different tools for healing.

The yoga, mindfulness, and Reiki chapters examine different ways you could adjust your personal practice to be more healing. Wherever you are in your trauma journey, there are adjustments you can make to support yourself. Even if you don't teach classes, you can apply these ideas to your own practices to support your well being.

Journal as you read through this book. From a personal angle, I find that writing down my thoughts helps me to go back later and see what has helped the most. Human memory is flawed. Having notes that tell me what benefited me in the past has always helped me during moments where I am struggling.

My thought processes

This book is designed to make you think. It isn't meant to be a reference dictionary that lays down the law of how to make trauma-informed recommendations. Instead, I want you to read this and apply the ideas I'm discussing. You may find certain therapies make sense for you. Other therapies may not resonate at this time. You may choose to reread this book in the future and it will speak to you in a totally different way.

I hope this book sparks discussion. I work with many people who have trauma, but that doesn't mean I have all the answers. Someone who specializes in different types of trauma will find situations that I haven't encountered.

For instance, one of my aromatherapy students brought up an interesting concern for clients who have experienced intimate partner violence. This student, Chaplain Nancy Lueschen, mentioned that she sees many of her clients struggle with woody scents. This may be because so many colognes have these scents as base notes. I never would have caught this myself, as I don't work exclusively with domestic violence situations.

As you can see, these conversations are already occurring. My students are frequently mentioning situations in which trauma-informed care could be tailored for their clients. Other practitioners have started talking about these issues. As I was finishing this book, two different virtual trauma-informed herbalism classes were hosted by other teachers. Our work is just beginning and I hope this book helps to guide you in your quest for better care.

We need more research

There needs to be more research done on trauma-informed care within natural practices. The information included in this book is mostly based on the experience of myself and other practitioners. Empirical evidence helps us to begin shaping trauma-informed practices, but research will help us to better understand what works best for most situations.

If we can create double blind, placebo controlled studies to show benefits of certain practices, we can shape our work to be more helpful. Codifying when therapies are most effective during stages of the trauma recovery process could make a world of difference. If you're a researcher, I encourage you to look into these things.

Conventional research doesn't always fit the paradigm of natural healthcare. Unless the doctor or professional designing the study has a background in holistic healthcare, there is usually too much focus on a conventional medicine diagnosis. Rarely does a research project consider constitutional analysis or specific symptom sets.

For instance, PTSD is a diagnosis that encompasses many different aspects of trauma-related anxiety. However, people who are suffering from PTSD may respond differently to different interventions based on their natural tendencies to be more tense or relaxed, hot or cold. When we can take these things into account, research results can completely change.

Forgive me, I digress. I just hope that those of you who have the ability to research these things further will do so.

Time to make a pledge

Consider making a promise. A promise to yourself, your family, community, and clients to become trauma-informed. Recognize how healing and connection can come through the appropriate application of natural remedies. Take time to learn what works for you, and for you practitioners take time to absorb even more that can help your clients.

Study how experiencing trauma can change our physiology. Understand that the trauma response is not a choice. Accept that healing can take time and lots of effort. Know that natural medicine is a wonderful way to help someone come into a safe, connected space that makes healing easier.

Discover how these physiological changes can cause us to respond differently to different modalities. Learn what plant medicines you resonate with most. Find other modalities that work for you. See how these things can help as we rewire ourselves and our clients for connection.

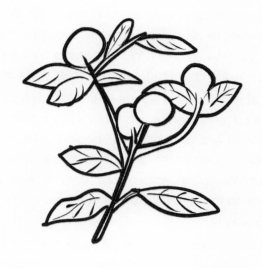

Chapter 2
Do No Harm

Herbalists set out on this path because of our strong connections to the Earth, her gifts, and the fascination with how powerful those gifts can be when correctly used. We usually come to this work because conventional medicine has failed us or someone close to us. We have witnessed how natural medicine can be life changing, when correctly applied.

One of the tenets of a healer is to do no harm. But *do no harm* is not a passive pledge: we have a responsibility to continue learning and growing. We should continue digging deeper, learning when herbs are contraindicated for certain energetic patterns and symptom sets. We can work to discover the exceptions to the rule so that we can help everyone in a personalized way.

We should also work to create a space in which we are not harming ourselves. Boundaries must be set, self care must be applied, and we must practice what we preach. Allowing ourselves to become overworked and not addressing emotions as they arise from secondary trauma can cause us to lose our way.

Our work to do no harm goes beyond what herbs are contraindicated in the physical body. Mental health is so important, and some conditions have symptoms that are exacerbated by the use of certain herbs. So why are we not looking deeper into trauma and how the different herbs and other healing techniques can be safely used?

Trauma care is becoming a popular topic. More and more people are saying they work with trauma, but when you begin digging into their history you realize they do not have proper training to adequately support clients with unresolved trauma. This is a major concern: when people are becoming retraumatized by untrained wellness practitioners, they may choose to never consider a natural approach again. Rightfully so - if your profession harms me, why should I return?

Some herbalists have begun looking at our work and have tried to see how we can be more effective when clients are struggling with trauma. Trauma-informed herbalists are starting to look deeper at how we can help someone who is struggling with plants and other complementary therapies. As a conscientious herbalist, you have picked up this book as part of an effort to understand better how to "do no harm". Hopefully the work I've done in putting together this resource will help you think further into the topic and come up with new ideas to improve the subject. Together we can help to make "trauma-informed" practice the norm instead of a novel idea.

Trauma-Informed is not a buzzword

"Trauma-informed" and "trauma sensitive" have become buzzwords. Their popularity is a double edged sword. I am grateful that it is becoming more common to recognize the need for trauma-informed care, but I see so many untrained healers offering "trauma-informed" support for clients with trauma.

"But I've been through so much myself! I understand what it is like to have trauma."

Yes, that sets us on the path toward wanting to help others who are struggling, but that is not the key to being trauma-informed. Our trauma experiences do not guarantee that we magically know how to address trauma in clients on a wider scale. This is a consistent theme throughout this book: good intentions do not absolve you of doing the deeper work.

I see the gaps in some of our sister healing modalities. Studios that are working to be more accessible may make certain classes quieter, scent-free, or with less bright lighting and label them "trauma sensitive" or "trauma-informed". But then you get into class and the teachers are using phrasing that is blatantly triggering or they do not appear to know what to do when a student begins to struggle.

I've seen people in many healing disciplines tout trauma sensitivity without any evidence indicating they have learned the psychology or physiology behind what occurs when someone suffers from trauma symptoms. Although they may have wonderful intentions, this is harmful. Best case scenario, a person is uncomfortable and decides that the class or healing option isn't for them. Worst case, the person is retraumatized and now has another layer of symptoms with which to struggle.

Trauma-informed is a pledge to do better

As a trauma-informed herbalist, you make a pledge to your clients to put them first during their consults. You promise to acknowledge their concerns and their experience without inserting your ideas or opinions. You will believe them when they say they are experiencing trauma.

You recognize the need to consistently be learning, growing, and revising your approach to caring for a client who is suffering from trauma. Trauma-informed best practices are in their infancy and will continue to morph as evidence shows what works best. I hope this book gets more people talking about trauma-informed care, and I hope in a decade I will have to rewrite this manuscript to include new cutting edge ideas and herbal therapies.

You also pledge to take care of yourself. You will treat yourself with gentleness and recognize that you also need support. We will discuss self care and self reflection in chapter seventeen, but go ahead and be thinking about how you could work to create a healthier environment for yourself.

Who needs trauma-informed care?

You may be asking, "how do I know who needs trauma-informed care?" The short answer: you don't really need to know at first. Your clients may not even know they have experienced trauma, much less that they need support.

I consider trauma-informed care part of my practice, not a separate piece. Instead of having one set of practices for non-trauma and another for trauma, I have built trauma-informed care into the systems I offer everyone. Therefore, I do not necessarily believe you have to know up front who has unresolved trauma in order to offer effective care.

In chapter four, we will discuss how to recognize when someone may be dealing with different types of trauma. This is for your edification, to help you to notice who might need more support. But we don't have to always know that someone is struggling (much less what they are struggling with) in order to offer safer practices.

While I do ask if someone has experienced trauma and give general examples to help them understand what I mean, I never ask for details about someone's trauma. If a person is comfortable they may share some details that help me shape their protocol, but I do not ask for specifics or try to dig into the experiences a person is sharing.

We don't want to make assumptions about how a person feels or what they have experienced, However, it isn't necessary for an herbalist to have all the specifics about a person's history. Pressing for specifics could cause a person to become uncomfortable, and possibly even retraumatized.

General trauma-informed protocols could include discussing the contents of a guided meditation before the class is led through the meditation, choosing language that is more inclusive and less likely to activate someone's trauma, or even adjusting the herbal protocols you offer to be less likely to exacerbate hyper- or hypo- arousal states.

Around half of the population will experience some form of traumatic event in their lifetime. The U.S. Department of Veterans Affairs suggests that 6% of the U.S. population will develop post traumatic stress disorder (PTSD) at some point in their lives[2]. More recent research suggests that these numbers may be significantly higher, with closer to 80% of humans experiencing a traumatic event and up to 10% of humans developing PTSD[3].

These numbers indicate that trauma-informed approaches to wellness are necessary. Many people are struggling with unresolved trauma, whether they have been diagnosed with PTSD or not. We can utilize some basic principles when working to be more trauma-informed in order to create a safer, more secure environment for everyone.

Trauma-informed care principles

Trauma-informed care offers a supportive way to help clients feel able to focus on their healing instead of spending their energy mitigating trauma symptoms. It helps to create an environment that is less likely to cause someone to become retraumatized. There are simple principles that can be implemented quickly for anyone who is interested in becoming more trauma-informed in their practice.

The University of Buffalo's Institute on Trauma and Trauma-Informed Care presents the idea of five trauma-informed care principles that can be applied to our work[1]. You will see elements of these principles throughout this book. Safety, choice, collaboration, trustworthiness, and empowerment are the five trauma-informed care principles that should govern your work.

Safety is the foundation on which the rest of our work is built. If a person does not feel a sense of physical and emotional safety in our presence, nothing else can be accomplished. We can do this by focusing on creating a trauma sensitive space and using trauma-informed language.

Choice is the initial offering that helps a person begin to trust their decision making process again. Offer clients choices around different treatment options instead of forcing a particular plan. However, also recognize that multiple choices can cause fatigue. There can even be times that choosing creates an immobilization response.

As with many aspects of trauma, everyone's response is different. Choices can be empowering for some, but others may find them overwhelming. When trauma occurs that takes away someone's ability to make choices, being presented with the opportunity to choose may feel like too much at first.

Offering the appropriate balance of choice and direction can be difficult. With many things in this book, it takes time and experience to find a harmonious solution. Start slow and offer tiny choices at first. Pay attention to your clients' body language and safely offer more choices as appropriate.

Collaboration is a portion of trauma-informed care that many herbalists already utilize. We recognize the need for our clients to be heard and respected. Collaborating with clients allows us to understand how they are feeling toward different recommendations. This principle is heavily intertwined with choice. When choice and collaboration are respected, it becomes easier for clients to develop a sense that you are a trustworthy ally.

Trustworthiness is an important part of trauma-informed care. Once a person has begun to place their trust in you as a facilitator on their healing journey, you must recognize the need to maintain a respectful relationship. Continue to enforce appropriate boundaries and always do your best to honor your word.

Boundaries can be a difficult thing when someone has been surrounded by unhealthy relationships. Many people with trauma may struggle to know what an appropriate boundary is in a professional relationship. Modeling good boundaries for clients can help them as they work to restructure their definition of what healthy relationships with others look like.

Empowerment is the final principle of trauma-informed care. Helping someone see their strengths and acknowledging when they do something well is an important key to helping a person with unresolved trauma. If you are practicing the first four principles, empowerment becomes much easier to successfully implement.

As you read through this book, keep these five principles in mind. How could you notice moments where these principles could help you with your inner work? How can you implement them in your day to day dealings with clients? Do you have ways you could work with your staff or other healers in the same space to apply these principles as a group?

Referring out

Trauma is complex. There are so many nuances to consider and individualized needs that you are not equipped to fulfill. Building a network of people who can help your clients leads them to a much better healing experience.

Today, I encourage you to go do some research on local options available to help people struggling with trauma. Having your clients visit other healers and professional medical providers is not a sign of weakness. It is a sign of a confident practitioner that knows when a person needs help from someone outside their realm of expertise.

Have a referral list that includes other natural practitioners, therapists who specialize in different types of trauma, and support groups. Different symptoms of trauma may benefit more from certain treatment options. Different traumatic incidents can be processed best with therapists and support groups that are designed to discuss the trauma that commonly occurs as part of those incidents.

Healing is easiest when a person is part of a community. In the modern digital age, this face to face interaction isn't as common. Sometimes people need support in finding their version of community. Do not hesitate to encourage people to find multiple avenues of healing and support. We will all benefit from stronger community connections.

In chapter eighteen, we will discuss referrals and working to connect to the healing community. However, do not wait until you've read this entire book before doing some research on options in your local area. You can go ahead and begin implementing these ideas now. You may even find an offering that can help you on your journey!

Commit to continuing education

As a trauma-informed herbalist, you must commit to continuing education. I know so many people who stopped attending other workshops and education opportunities because they felt they had learned enough to be effective. Less than five years later, they are offering outdated advice that has been replaced with a more effective system and clients are suffering because of it.

The trauma-informed approach to herbalism (and other natural therapies) is still in its infancy. Do not read this book once, check off a mark on your to-do list, and consider your education in trauma-informed care complete. Take a class in trauma-informed care. Read books on trauma and its effects on the body. Work to learn under a trauma-informed teacher. There is so much more to learn and so many more things to discover. Your work is just beginning.

As I mentioned in the introduction, many of the discussions around herbal protocols are still in the theory/hypothesis stage. My anecdotal evidence shows that we can confidently continue to work with these methods and attempt to refine the trauma-informed protocols… and my main reason for writing this book is to share my work in hopes that you will join me on this quest. Part of your pledge is to take this information, expand upon it, and grow this field so that we can help people with even more effective natural therapies!

Continuing education can also create a chance to look at the adaptability of the protocols you have in place. The more you learn about your chosen modalities, the easier it will be to adapt them to someone's needs. The skill of noticing how you could adapt and working to support your clients goes beyond trauma-informed care: it is a trait that sets the most successful practitioners apart from their less conscientious colleagues.

Supporting under-represented communities

One final point that I would like to address from the angle of doing no harm: we must consider how to shape our offerings so that people in under-represented communities also have access. Herbalism used to be the medicine of the people. In many ways, it still is. However, many aspects have been gentrified.

Our capitalistic society encourages the commodification of wellness. Trauma-informed herbalists must recognize how the systems in place are inherently discriminatory. Many people who could benefit from our work cannot access healing because of issues such as financial struggle, limited transportation, and access to childcare. There are other people who may not feel comfortable working with you and may need access to someone who understands their culture.

Sliding scale offerings are becoming more common in the natural health community. Suggested rates are usually based on salary, financial commitments and debt, and disability. Play with how you offer this. You may find certain systems work best for you and your clients.

I love Leanne Holcomb's sliding scale offering through her business, One Tree Healing Arts. She offers a chart detailing the recommended appointment fee based on your annual salary. However, she also adds that an annual salary is not a complete picture of someone's financial security. People may choose to shift up or down the fee scale based on financial assets or debts that could change their ability to afford a session. She also makes it clear that she does not ask you how you arrived at the amount you pay.

Her sliding scale is well thought out and fits the pledge of a trauma-informed herbalist. She offers a clear range of fees, offers suggestions on how to choose the best fee, and guarantees that you will not encounter derision for your choice.

It's a fantastic example of how we can be conscientious and still be compensated fairly for the work we are doing.

There are many other ways we can make our work more accessible. Sometimes scholarships and pro bono work are warranted. Sometimes we should work to change the way we present an offering to accommodate a person who has a disability. Think proactively about ways you could help others gain access to your work.

Sometimes it isn't about getting access to you; sometimes people need to know where they could access practitioners with similar cultural beliefs or values. Amplifying the voices of people who have been disenfranchised is an important part of making sure our work is accessible for everyone. We will talk more in chapter nineteen about things to consider when working to support marginalized groups.

Final thoughts

As you continue into this book, notice how your pledge to do no harm as a trauma-informed herbalist can come into play. Notice suggestions that could help you implement principles such as choice, collaboration, trustworthiness, healthy boundaries, and empowerment. After you've finished your first read through, come back to this chapter and notice if anything new sticks out to you.

In the next chapter, we begin exploring how trauma changes a person. I present this information in order to help you see why it can be so difficult for a person to heal. It is rarely as simple as learning how to "just relax" or "tough it out". There are several moving parts to trauma and only a holistic approach is going to offer the fastest, most effective relief.

References

1. *What is trauma-informed care?* University at Buffalo School of Social Work - University at Buffalo. (2022, March 31). Retrieved May 30, 2022, from https://socialwork.buffalo.edu/social-research/institutes-centers/institute-on-trauma-and-trauma-informed-care/what-is-trauma-informed-care

2. *Va.gov: Veterans Affairs*. How Common is PTSD in Adults? (2018, September 13). Retrieved March 12, 2022, from https://www.ptsd.va.gov/understand/common/common_adults.asp

3. Mann, S. K., & Marwaha, R. (2022). Posttraumatic Stress Disorder. In *StatPearls*. StatPearls Publishing.

Chapter 3
How Trauma Changes Us

What is trauma?

Dr. Bessel van der Kolk states that trauma is the response of the body to an event that is (consciously or subconsciously) perceived as unbearable or intolerable[1]. Notice, he states it is the reaction of the body - not the event itself.

Individuals may respond to a variety of stressors in a multitude of ways. Unresolved trauma symptoms vary widely. No particular response is "right". Certain responses do not indicate that the person is "weaker" than someone else.

As trauma-informed herbalists, it is important for us to hold space for clients as they share their trauma situations. Science is showing us that trauma's existence is not based on whether or not a person was tough enough. It's not a matter of trying to "suck it up". Trauma is a real and normal reaction that the body has - regardless of how smart, brave, or strong a person is.

Wired for fear, wired for connection

We are about to discuss theories that dive deeper into the trauma response, how the body stores trauma, and how different options may be available to release trauma. But do not be overwhelmed! I want you to explore a deeper understanding of the trauma response, but if you remember nothing else, remember the phrase: "Wired for fear or wired for connection".

This phrase embodies the idea that people immediately react to situations by either being afraid or by reaching for connection. When someone is "wired for fear", they're not *choosing* to be fearful. Instead, this is a survival mechanism that has occurred and they are now stuck in that reaction. Their body and brain are attempting to keep them safe, which results in a distorted response from the nervous system.

The solution to an overactive "wired for fear" response is to consciously rewire the system to be more "wired for connection". Rewiring can be a slow, complex process. Usually there are many wires criss-crossed and there isn't an immediate fix. If you've ever seen a computer server room that has been haphazardly put together, you can envision how this process will take time. The only way to approach this is with patience, understanding, and acknowledgement of slow, steady progress over a period of time

We see physical echoes of this wiring in certain forms of trauma through MRI scans of the brain. Many types of trauma that lead to a diagnosis of PTSD are linked to a reduction in gray matter[2]. The areas that suffer from gray matter reduction are specific to the type of trauma a person experiences.

Gestational environments, early childhood experiences, and epigenetics can have us predisposed to being wired for fear. However, the body's response is more complex than this. Even if we're lucky enough to experience a childhood that wires us for connection, events that occur later in life can cause us to rewire for fear. As trauma-informed herbalists, we play an important role as part of a team that helps clients to bring their system out of fear and back to connection in the face of stressors.

The nervous system's connection to trauma

The nervous system is extremely important in trauma related responses. This system has many moving parts that can all be affected by trauma. As with many subjects we will discuss, we could spend a whole separate book diving into the nervous system alone.

The nervous system can be divided into the central and peripheral nervous system. There are two functional systems within the peripheral nervous system that we will discuss here. The first is the somatic nervous system. The second is the autonomic nervous system.

The somatic nervous system controls our conscious movement. The brain sends impulses down and into our muscles to encourage movement through this system. When you decide to brush your hair or kick a soccer ball, your somatic system has helped you achieve that.

The autonomic nervous system is its "sister system" that controls involuntary or subconscious processes in the body. Frequently, the autonomic nervous system is the part of the nervous system most obviously disrupted when trauma sets into the body. The autonomic system is made up of the sympathetic and parasympathetic systems.

The sympathetic nervous system is the part of our system that helps us to be alert. When trauma over activates the response of the sympathetic nervous system, the "fight" or "flight" mechanisms are triggered. Trauma responses can cause the sympathetic nervous system to become easily excited, leading a person into a hyperarousal state.

The parasympathetic nervous system is the part of our system that helps us to "rest and digest". Sometimes trauma responses activate the parasympathetic system and can lead to a "freeze" response. This response can become extreme, even leading a person to become unconscious. Unresolved trauma can cause the parasympathetic nervous system to be triggered at the first sign of stress, causing someone to experience hypoarousal.

Once these responses become hardwired into our system, the brain begins to recognize them as a useful tool to keep us safe when a future situation seems dangerous. The reaction occurs without giving us a chance to decide how we *want* to respond. This is important to understand: trauma responses are ingrained reactions that someone cannot will away. It takes time and concerted effort to change these survival reactions. These efforts are most effective when they address the mental, emotional, physical, and subtle energy layers of the body.

The Polyvagal Theory

Stephen Porges' Polyvagal Theory helps to shape our understanding of how the autonomic nervous system responds to traumatic events. The reactions described in polyvagal theory are predictable and are based on an hierarchical understanding of how the nervous system has developed. This theory helps to explain why safe social interactions and coregulation through group activities can be so helpful during one's trauma healing journey.

As mentioned above, there are two primary defense mechanisms that occur when a person encounters a dangerous situation. There is either a "fight or flight" response or the "freeze" response. In polyvagal theory, this fight or flight response is from the sympathetic nervous system. The freeze, or immobilization response, comes from the dorsal vagal system. However, there is a third system, the ventral vagal system, that helps to regulate the two survival responses.

The ventral part of the vagus nerve is directly connected with signals that control facial expression, vocal sounds, and head movement. This ventral vagal system allows for social engagement and coregulation. Safe interactions with people allow us to downregulate the defense responses and enter a space of relaxation and connection. It can interact with the dorsal vagal system to create a state of healthy intimacy. The ventral vagal system also interacts with the sympathetic system to allow for a state of play.

When a person experiences a traumatic event, this ventral vagal system can "go offline" and cause a person to not be able to return to a state of feeling safe and secure. This causes the dorsal vagal and sympathetic systems to run rampant. It can cause disruption to the neuroception processes that naturally occur.

Neuroception helps us to interpret signals we are experiencing to determine if we are safe and secure. When someone has unresolved trauma, interoception (what we feel internally) and exteroception (what we feel in regards to external stimuli) experiences are out of sync. So when a traumatized person experiences something that would commonly be considered benign, their body reacts to the experience as if it detected dangerous stimuli.

Top down and bottom up processing

Working to resolve trauma usually comes in the form of processing the body's reaction through "top down" or "bottom up" processing. These directional descriptors come from the "triune brain" theory that says the brain has three layers that process information. These three layers are the reptilian brain (the instinctual, survival center), the paleomammalian brain (the limbic, emotional center), and the neomammalian brain (the logical, abstract center).

Top down processing engages the mammalian brain in a type of logical processing that helps integrate things through language and abstract thinking. Bottom-up processing focuses on a reptilian brain through somatic experiences that help integrate things through sensations that arise from emotion. Both forms of processing trauma are valid, though they appear to be more beneficial at different times in the healing process.

Talk therapy tends to consist heavily of a top down processing approach. Cognitive behavioral therapy is an example of a commonly used top down processing therapy. It appears to work best once a person is able to feel regulated and safe. Many people find that top down processing is difficult in the early days of the trauma healing journey because the ventral vagal system is dormant.

Bottom up processing is a better option for people who are still stuck in their survival response state. Somatic experiencing techniques are examples of bottom up processing. Many people respond well to a somatic experiencing approach, especially early on in their healing journey. Many movement therapies support some form of bottom up processing. I speak more on somatic experiencing in chapter fourteen.

As trauma-informed herbalists, we are not looking to process trauma. However, we can consider how we approach someone to reach them in their state of survival. For instance, we can use a bottom up approach by softening our body language and using a soothing tone of voice that can help to calm the reptilian brain.

Repressing emotions

Social expectations on how emotions are handled can be passed on without anyone ever explaining these expectations. The first funeral I remember was my step-great grandfather's. He was a favorite of mine and I was horrified that Mac was gone. I wasn't five years old yet, but I could tell by the actions of everyone around me that I shouldn't cry. I suppressed all the grief I felt, barely able to breathe as the funeral progressed. When I got home, I locked the door and hid under my bed to sob for what felt like hours.

Our current culture has created a perfect storm for unresolved trauma to fester. We avoid displays of emotions that are deemed "negative". This repression has taught us that feeling strong emotions is a dangerous thing. Many times we may find ourselves unable to express emotions and these suppressions can cause us to be more susceptible to symptoms of unresolved trauma.

With the recent pandemic, I believe we are seeing the result of our culture's refusal to face negative emotions. I have heard so many more stories of adults acting out and pitching fits toward retail workers. I've witnessed colleagues become disheartened by the unprofessional behavior of others. This seems to be coming from the heightened state of stress that everyone is experiencing. The problem is exacerbated by the fact that most people don't understand how to remain mindful, neutral observers in the face of stress. We have not been taught how to manage hard feelings, much less how to help the body complete the stress cycle.

The stress cycle

When we experience a dangerous situation, our body reacts to keep us safe. When the natural progression of this protective reaction is disrupted, a person's nervous system may not fully reset. If we've experienced a disruption of the stress cycle, unresolved trauma symptoms may occur.

These symptoms vary widely, but are usually set off by events that make us feel similar to the original traumatic event. The circumstances of these events could be totally different (and usually the event is a benign situation), but our body reacts as if the threat has returned. Many people try to stuff these sensations away and carry on as before.

Trying to repress these negative feelings can have significant consequences. Many people struggle with physical symptoms that arise due to the stress. The negative feelings may cause a person to avoid situations that set them off. The longer these sensations are repressed, the more seemingly unrelated symptoms may bubble to the surface.

If we can learn how to complete the stress cycle, we can find ourselves less likely to suffer from unresolved trauma symptoms. Drs. Amelia and Emily Nagoski have written a book called Burnout: The Secret to Unlocking the Stress Cycle. While the book is not focused directly on trauma, it is a discussion around stress and has a lot of practical advice for processing stressful situations.

Creativity, affection from a safe person or animal, breathwork, physical exercise, and emotional expression are all ways we can work to complete the stress cycle. Different activities may support one person better than another. We can help clients learn what ways they can support a reduced stress response in their body.

When a person does not know they can consciously work to reduce their stress response, they become more susceptible to a trauma reaction. The buildup of stress can lead a person to feel worn down. This can lead to a narrowing of the window of tolerance, making it hard for a person to fully recover.

The window of tolerance

Dr. Dan Siegel's window of tolerance helps to illustrate the space a person is in when they are feeling able to safely interact with their environment. A person is in their window of tolerance when they are able to be present in the moment with an appropriate reaction from their body. The ability to experience empathy and be open and curious to new experiences is a sign someone is in their window of tolerance.

Hyperarousal occurs when we feel amplified above and beyond the window of tolerance. A sense of intense energy and a need to defend oneself is common. Racing thoughts, anger, and becoming engulfed in an emotional response can occur. Feeling "tensed up" in a fight or flight reaction indicates hyperarousal.

Hypoarousal occurs when we drop below the window of tolerance. A sense of disconnect and depletion of energy is common. A numbing, passive response can occur when someone is in a hyperarousal state. Freeze responses are indications of hypoarousal.

When we experience trauma, our window of tolerance can start to narrow. We may find ourselves unable to abide the same level of stress as before. Even good sources of stress, sometimes called eustress, may feel intolerable. Certain activities may no longer be enjoyable because they feel overstimulating.

The window of tolerance can be expanded, with the right therapeutic practices. As an herbalist, most of these practices are not within your scope. However, we can help a person become more aware of when they are in their window of tolerance. We can also help people become more aware of the activities that help them complete the stress cycle and stay in their window of tolerance. We will also discuss nervine herbs in chapter nine that could reduce an overactive nervous system and help a person feel their window of tolerance has expanded.

The window of tolerance is a helpful visualization for anyone when they are under stress. It is especially useful when a person has struggled with some form of trauma. Using this imagery can help people become more self aware and realize what helps them the most.

Acute trauma

There are many ways to describe the experience of trauma and its pervasiveness in our world today. One way is to look at the time frame of the trauma that occurs. Acute, chronic, and complex trauma are different ways we can see how trauma occurs and the reactions it can shape in a person.

These categorizations should only be used to help us identify how a person might experience trauma. Keep in mind that every person is different. Acute traumas are not necessarily more traumatizing than an ongoing chronic trauma. Some complex trauma clients are not going to respond the same as others. We cannot group people's reactions into their types of trauma, but understanding different types can help us see how many people may be unconsciously living with unresolved trauma.

Acute trauma is a short lived event that is terrifying and is usually easily recognized as trauma by society. Usually the events directly related to acute trauma last less than a few weeks. Witnessing a death, being in a car crash, living through a natural disaster, or experiencing a terrorist attack are all forms of acute trauma.

Chronic trauma

Chronic trauma is an ongoing event that affects a person multiple times. Whereas an acute trauma is usually a singular event with a clear moment of trauma, chronic trauma can continue to traumatize a person over a long period of time. Many types of chronic trauma may not be obvious to us from a cursory glance. Many types of chronic trauma are not obvious even to those who have suffered through them.

Exposure to systemic discrimination, long term illness, domestic abuse, adoption, living in an unsafe community, and food insecurity are just a few examples of stressors that can create chronic trauma. These events can leave a person feeling disconnected, unsure of who is safe, and feeling as if a trustworthy community does not exist for them. Chronic traumas tend to cause more subtle, long-lasting effects. A person may not equate these chronic traumas as the root of emotional and physical suffering they consequently experience.

Complex trauma

Complex trauma creates another dimension to trauma-informed care. Trauma is seen as "complex" when a person is exposed to a variety of different types of trauma, creating a complex response. While chronic trauma is a different classification from complex trauma, chronic trauma can easily become complex.

We've spoken about the "fight or flight" and "freeze" responses to trauma. Another commonly discussed reaction is known as the "fawn" response. This response mainly occurs in victims of complex trauma. Someone may have discovered that people pleasing and disconnecting from their own thoughts and emotions is the easiest way to avoid dangerous situations they are accustomed to experiencing. The brain realizes this fawning is keeping them safe, and it begins to default to this response anytime it detects danger.

The fawn response may make it more difficult for a person to contradict a person in authority. When you are working with someone that has complex trauma, pay particular attention to your suggestions and questions. We can inadvertently guide someone toward agreeing with us if we are not careful. Instead of asking leading questions or making statements hinting at the answer you are looking for, work to offer a more neutral communication. Neutral discussions allow our clients who have a tendency toward "fawn" to express their needs more clearly.

Acute, chronic, and complex trauma situations are becoming more pervasive. We must recognize that there are many people who are struggling with unresolved trauma - consciously or unconsciously. In the next chapter, we will explore different ways we may become aware that someone is struggling with trauma. We will also discuss what to do if a person begins struggling when they are with us.

References

1. Van der Kolk, B. (2015). *The Body Keeps the Score: Brain, Mind, and Body in the Healing of Trauma*. Penguin Publishing.

2. Meng L, Jiang J, Jin C, Liu J, Zhao Y, Wang W, Li K, Gong Q. Trauma-specific Grey Matter Alterations in PTSD. Sci Rep. 2016 Sep 21;6:33748. doi: 10.1038/srep33748. PMID: 27651030; PMCID: PMC5030628.

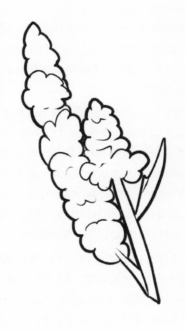

Chapter 4
Recognizing Trauma

Unresolved trauma shows up in a variety of ways. Many people may not have a diagnosis that points to trauma as the source of their struggles. They may not even be aware that part of their health concerns stem from a traumatic event. Everyone's situation is different and we have to be ready to act according to their needs.

We do not have to have all the details of someone's trauma to be helpful. If they choose to share their experience with us, we should listen and help them feel heard. However, I never ask for details about a client's trauma. We are not trained to process trauma with clients. Asking questions risks them beginning to feel outside their window of tolerance or feeling pressured to share more than they wanted.

So if we are not digging into the narrative around someone's trauma response, how do we know what will help people? We have a variety of tools at our disposal for becoming aware of trauma's effects in someone's life. We can encourage self regulation, look toward making our work more trauma sensitive, and implement appropriate herbal interventions.

As trauma-informed herbalists, we can ask clients if they have been struggling with stressful events. That may help us see how trauma has played a role in our clients' health and wellbeing. We can also notice signs and symptoms that may present without a person knowing they are related to trauma.

No matter where we find people on their healing journey, we work to find appropriate ways to support them without retraumatization. We can adjust our protocols to be helpful for anyone's needs if we educate ourselves enough. Once we are able to recognize the effects of trauma, we can be more effective at our recommendations and support systems.

No diagnosis necessary

Many people who struggle with trauma may not have an official diagnosis. They may not have symptoms that fit neatly into the DSM-5's description of trauma related disorders. Their symptoms may not be severe enough to warrant a diagnosis, but can still have a significant impact on their well being. Many people may not have the official diagnosis, but they could still benefit from trauma-informed care.

You may find some clients who are hesitant to work with a therapist or psychiatrist. I regularly encounter people who do not trust conventional medical care and are hesitant to work with mental health professionals. Many people equate mental health care with snake oil medicine.

There are also those that feel that seeking help from mental health professionals is a dangerous thing. Some equate mental healthcare to rejecting their faithfully held religious beliefs. They may have hesitancy because admitting they need psychological help could indicate to their community that their salvation is at risk.

People in BIPOC communities may hesitate to seek care because of the way public health has betrayed them in the past. These health related abuses were not that long ago: the Tuskegee experiments occurred in our grandparents' generation. It is understandable that these experiences still cause concern.

We can work to find ways to introduce hesitant people to safe, reliable counselors and therapists, but I digress. Whatever the situation, a diagnosis of PTSD or other trauma related illness may not be available. That is alright. As trauma-informed herbalists, we recognize a medical diagnosis is not a prerequisite for offering trauma sensitive care.

If someone does have a diagnosis, that helps us recognize they may need trauma-informed care. However, there are many different ways a trauma related diagnosis can present. We do not treat physical disease based on diagnoses, neither should we address mental disease based on a diagnosis. As always, herbalists should be paying attention to the signs and symptoms of unresolved trauma manifesting in a person. These indicators can help us make a plan specific to the individual's needs.

Ask during intake

My intake form asks people if they have a history of any traumatic events in their past. I phrase this question as a yes or no question on my intake, not asking for details. I find the people who want you to have details will explain further.

"Trauma" is a word that many people still equate with very specific types of events. If you ask this question, I encourage you to list out a few examples of different types of trauma. Especially things people might not normally equate with their traumatic effects such as living in an unsafe community, multiple medical procedures, or witnessing another person's trauma.

I also ask if people have any current stressors that are making things difficult for them. A follow up question to this is if they have any past stressors that are still causing them distress. Many people will admit to certain "stresses" in their life that you and I might call trauma - even if they do not label them as such.

My final question in this section of my intake is to have clients rate different possible sources of stress for them. On a scale of 1 (none at all) to 5 (overwhelming), I ask them to say how stressful certain aspects of their life feel. I include school, work, family, and health, among other things. This doesn't directly screen for trauma, but it can help me see a more holistic picture of where they may be struggling.

On my intake form I also ask about professionals a person is currently seeing. This can sometimes reveal they are working with a therapist or counselor. I cannot assume that they are in therapy for trauma, but it may be a context clue that points to the need to be more trauma sensitive with my client.

Asking is not foolproof. Some people will still not necessarily want to claim their difficult situations as traumatic. They may justify the events as "just a part of life." Other people may not feel comfortable revealing they are seeing a therapist or counselor. As trauma-informed herbalists, we do not judge the decision to tell us or not tell us these things. We just use the information presented to help us make a better plan for our clients.

When a client tells you they've experienced trauma

Believe clients when they tell you they have experienced trauma. Someone may seem perfectly functional, but you do not know what they've done in order to make sure they could show up to their appointment with you. They may have sacrificed all other activities for that day to make sure they had the energy to control their symptoms while working with you.

Normally asking questions is a sign of empathy, but in the case of trauma it can actually cause someone to struggle. Probing questions can cause a person to feel that they need to justify their trauma to you. They may also feel that you do not believe them.

Instead of asking questions, validate the person's feelings. "I can see how hard that must have been," or "Thank you for sharing, that sounds tough," can help someone feel heard. Do not say "I know how you feel." Even if you have a similar experience, it is not an appropriate response to help someone feel validated.

If a client's situation sounds ludicrous to you, do not try to offer advice or try to logically explain how it could have been different. As trauma-informed herbalists, we are not here to tell someone what they should have done, could have done, or what we would have done in their place. Instead, we can take the opportunity to reinforce the fact that their body did exactly what it needed to do to survive - that the response they had was a sign of their body taking care of them in that moment.

Self awareness of the effects of stress

If a person acknowledges they have significant stress or trauma in their life, I like to find out if they notice anything that can activate their stress. If a person is already aware of certain things that make their stress worse, it can help jumpstart my recommendations. Many people come to me already somewhat aware of their body's needs. They can tell me what foods cause distress, what activities are difficult, and some can even identify certain TV show genres that are activating for them. If I know what makes stress worse, we can determine what interventions we will avoid.

I also want to know what makes stress better. Do they have a workout plan that helps them feel more grounded afterward? Are there certain people or pets that help them co-regulate? What are people doing to manage stress as it occurs? If they have these answers, it may help us to make a plan in case they begin to feel bad during a session.

Although clients making these observations is helpful, it is not a requirement for building an effective plan. As trauma-informed herbalists, we do not pass judgment if someone is unsure of what might be best for them. Even joking comments like "in this day and age, how do you not have a plan to manage stress?" could hurt. We can inadvertently create a barrier by making comments that could be misconstrued as hurtful.

In later chapters, we will discuss ways that we can help someone become more mindfully aware of what works for them physically and emotionally. When someone comes to us without much self awareness, we have a chance to help them find their gameplan. Do not risk the trust you are building with a glib remark.

Signs of trauma activation

When a client first walks in, I take note of their energy, their tone of voice, and their body language. This helps me to determine aspects of their constitution, but it also helps me recognize when something changes during our session. Someone who comes in loud and with big movements could go quiet when asked about something that makes them uncomfortable. Someone with good eye contact may lose that eye contact when asked about something that makes them feel shame.

If someone begins fidgeting, biting or picking at their fingernails, or bouncing their leg up and down during a session, that can be a sign that they're attempting to self soothe. They may start holding their breath or stiffen their body. They may become distant and struggle to pay attention to the questions you are asking.

Physical indicators of discomfort do not automatically mean someone is dealing with unresolved trauma. However, noticing someone's response alongside other signs we have detailed in this chapter may help you hone in on how to best address concerns. If someone becomes too uncomfortable, they can leave their window of tolerance and become hyper- or hypo- aroused.

Remember hyperarousal and hypoarousal from the last chapter? When someone leaves their window of tolerance and begins experiencing a survival response, they may describe symptoms of these states of arousal. Understanding a bit about what occurs lets us be more aware of what our clients may be experiencing.

Hyperarousal can cause feelings of irritability, anger, or panic. Someone who is in a state of hyperarousal is usually jittery and will be easily startled. Your clients may find their focus being quickly pulled from one thing to the next. A person who is struggling with hyperarousal may describe it as a sense of always being on alert or needing to plan for the worst.

Hypo arousal seems to be less common, but can be just as disorienting for a person who is struggling with trauma. The sensation is almost like shutting down. A person may become numb or spaced out. Drowsiness can occur and your clients may mention it feels like they struggle to be able to respond.

What to do if a client is struggling

What if a client begins having a panic attack during a session? What if symptoms of hypo- or hyper- arousal occur? The best thing you can do is stay calm and help them come back into their body. If a client begins struggling, I work to help them ground and then we determine whether or not they want to continue or reschedule. What the client has mentioned helped them previously may determine what works best for us in these moments.

If someone begins struggling, stay calm and remain empathetic. Try not to say things such as "take it easy" or "calm down". Because someone may be moving into a reptilian brain response state, logical discussion won't help much. If you've asked in advance, you should have some idea as to what type of activity helps them.

Some people like to keep talking and others may prefer to sit in silence. Some people want to stay seated, others may need to get up and walk for a few minutes before returning to their seat for calm breathing. Someone may like to reach for a sudoku puzzle while someone else may do best to listen to music for a few moments.

If dysregulation occurs, stay with your client until they are coming back into a state of focused awareness. Work with them to determine if you should continue the session or reschedule. Always have them follow up with their therapist and encourage them to continue looking for self-regulating exercises to help them in moments of distress.

You may want to try some of the exercises below and see what helps you. You might create a handout of a few self-regulating exercises for your clients to try. Educating people about ways to self-regulate can help in moments where they are struggling, but do not forget that you should also encourage them to find a therapist to help them process their trauma.

Self regulation exercises

One exercise I like to use to help myself ground is designed to redirect us to our most tangible senses. You slowly name five things you see, four things you hear, three things you can touch, two things you can smell, and one thing you can taste. Focus for a few seconds on each item, paying attention to the sense it activates. This can help you to come back into your body and refocus on the present moment.

Slow breathing exercises help most people who are in a hyperarousal state. Box breathing is a common exercise that can be useful. For box breathing, you count as you breathe.

For instance, inhale, counting to four.

Hold the breath, counting to four.

Exhale, counting to four.

Hold, counting to four, and then repeat.

Sometimes I find it helpful to create a longer exhale, counting to six on exhale and not holding at the bottom of the breath for as long. These longer exhales can help to activate the ventral vagal system, quickly bringing us back to a feeling of safety.

Be aware that a few people may feel more activated when drawn to their breath. Medical incidents, domestic violence, and even racial discrimination experiences may cause a person to feel more anxious around their breath. Get to know someone before suggesting breathing exercises during times of vulnerability. I talk more about breathing in the context of mindfulness and meditation in chapter thirteen.

Sometimes distraction helps. Noticing a part of the body that feels safe and bringing focus to it can be helpful for someone who is no longer in their window of tolerance. This exercise felt silly to me at first, because it was only a small portion of my body that felt safe: maybe a pinky or my kneecap. What I found was the longer I practiced this, the easier it was to find a sense of safety in larger areas. Focusing on the feeling of safety that is found in a part of the body during hyper- or hypo-arousal can help you re-enter that window of tolerance.

Bilateral stimulation devices may be an option for some people. These devices make a buzzing sensation, alternating from one side to the other. I have bilateral stimulation bracelets that I love to wear. I have also recently bought a device that offers more options of buzz frequency and strength. Although they are relatively expensive, these devices can help to stop the catastrophizing that can sometimes cause a person to begin to struggle.

There are many self regulation exercises available. I encourage you to do some research and see what other exercises might work for you and your clients. These self regulation exercises are mostly symptom management. Encouraging clients to work with a therapist can help them to get healing at the root cause.

Everyone is different

We're discussing theories and research in this book that can help better support you, your family, and your clients. However, everyone is going to present differently, respond differently, and find different tools useful. As a trauma-informed herbalist, you have the responsibility to recognize this and plan accordingly.

In the next few chapters, we are going to discuss trauma-informed language, trauma sensitive spaces, and your scope of practice. When you are reading through this information, recognize that not everything is going to matter for you and your clients. You may reread this book in a few years and find that new things stick out that matter more compared to now. Take what works for you, implement it, and study further to understand what will help the most.

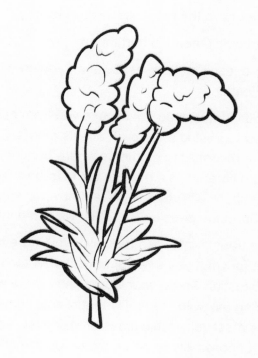

Chapter 5
Trauma Informed
Language

Words have the power to heal or destroy.

"But I didn't mean to hurt them!"

This doesn't matter - especially if you aren't making an effort to get better.

Good intentions do not excuse you from becoming more aware of your phrasing and how it affects others. Exercising empathy and recognizing moments where our choice of words can make a difference is a mark of being trauma-informed. We all have a responsibility to recognize that what we say can support or harm the people with which we come into contact.

As a trauma-informed herbalist, you are even more responsible for what you say. Your position of authority places you into a situation where your words carry more weight. Compounding this with the reality that clients come to you in some of the most vulnerable times of their lives: you have a significant responsibility to weigh the phrases that you choose.

If you are of a group of people that has some form of advantage in our society, you also hold another level of power that can cause your words to cut even further. If you're white, male, cisgendered, or heterosexual, you need to take more time to recognize how you may be blind to the struggles of marginalized groups. As a cisgendered white person, I recognize there are experiences I will never fully understand. With this knowledge, I work to change my behavior to be more accepting and supportive.

I mess up. I try to find opportunities to learn and I have trusted friends and colleagues to help me reexamine my actions when I find myself lacking. As a trauma-informed herbalist, I encourage you to find people in your life you trust to tell you the truth and speak from a place of kindness.

Eating disorders and weight

There are several situations in which paying attention to trauma-informed language can make a significant difference in the way a client feels. First off, let's explore eating disorders. People with trauma will sometimes find themselves facing an eating disorder as they attempt to survive the feelings and experiences they are facing. This means you may encounter clients with eating disorders frequently as a trauma-informed practitioner.

Let me take you back to one of my first interactions that caused me to second guess whether my training was adequate for the real world situations my clients faced. At the time, I was not screening for eating disorders (or any significant trauma situations).

We were discussing water intake. Martha didn't drink enough water, and needed guidelines as to how much to drink per day. I had been taught that the appropriate recommendation was half of someone's body weight, in ounces.

So, as was tradition, I asked "How much do you weigh?"

"I don't know, and I don't want to know. I've struggled with eating disorders my entire life," Martha replied.

Oops. I messed that one up...

"Ah, OK, let's stick with 60-80 ounces of water per day and see how you feel. We can adjust at our next session"

"Sounds good," she said, and we continued on with our session.

Martha was gracious about the interaction, but it was a stinging reminder of what I was discovering: we build many of our protocols without considering the struggles that many people face. How nerve wracking that conversation could be for some people! I could have easily triggered someone unintentionally with that discussion. I now screen for eating disorders in my intake paperwork and do not ask about weight if someone discloses they have struggled with them in the past.

Speaking of weight, how an herbalist discusses someone's weight can completely change the way a person feels about their experience. Paying attention to bias and not dismissing someone just because they do not fit an ideal is extremely important for a trauma-informed herbalist. Whether over- or under- weight, a person who is struggling with weight can feel stressed about working with a practitioner.

It's become common knowledge in the past few years that obese patients are treated very differently. Doctors may view obese patients as non-compliant, lazy, or dumb. This leads practitioners to dismiss treatment resistant symptoms, assume a person's health issues are exclusively related to weight, and not take health concerns seriously.

Weight issues of any kind can exacerbate trauma responses and cause people to be uncomfortable and hyper aroused in any sort of clinic setting. Clients may come to you hesitant because of trauma around the way they've been treated by other health professionals. Being aware of the biases against people with weight concerns can help you avoid falling into those traps yourself.

Gender

Similarly to weight bias, women can find themselves struggling to be heard by practitioners. I have been in multiple medical situations where it became clear that I was not being taken seriously because of my gender. Many women worry that someday they will be experiencing dangerous symptoms and no doctor will believe them.

Because of the patriarchal leaning of our society, everyone should take stock of how they feel toward women. Even women may find themselves believing damaging stereotypes about their gender. Make sure that the language you are using is gender inclusive and does not have undertones of negative stereotypes.

On the topic of gender and sexuality, be aware of the way you speak about these topics in general. Many people are not comfortable speaking out about their sexuality and their journey. If they begin to realize you are an ally, they are more likely to be willing to open up and work with you. This means you would be able to offer them more personalized support on their health journey.

My friend Catherine has recently begun hormone treatment for her transition. One of the things that has struck me is how much it meant to her when she came out at work and everyone quickly accepted her real pronouns and began calling her by her correct name. She speaks of this experience with a slight tremble in her voice, clearly ecstatic by the fact that everyone chose to be affirming.

Does using affirming language and addressing someone with their correct pronouns completely fix the systemic discrimination that occurs for people in the LGBTQ+ community? No: it would be completely reductionist to allude to such a notion. Do these actions move us toward creating a safe, healing space for our clients to feel supported? The hope is yes.

My intake form now has a blank space for pronouns instead of a limiting multiple choice of he/him, she/her, they/them. I encourage you to go ahead and change your intake to something similar; I'm proud to report that, even here in the Deep South, I have yet to have someone mock that option or abuse it in any way. All it has done is help people, who just want to disclose their unique pronouns in a safe way, communicate that to me.

Race

Another tragically common language issue surrounds race oppression. There are myriads of racially charged phrases such as "peanut gallery", Master bed/bathroom, "grandfathered in", and "gypped". These phrases come from attempts at dehumanizing and criminalizing minorities.

Also, notice where you may borrow phrases or language from a culture that is not your own. In some situations, this is appropriate. Other times, it is appropriation. Be mindful and listen to what people from that culture say about the phrasing and its history.

You will not always be aware of the history of phrases, but there are people educating us on these offensive word choices all the time. If you have trusted friends that are more in tune with racially charged language, ask them to send you two or three of their favorite articles on the subject. The more cognizant you are of racially or ethnically charged statements, the better equipped you are to support people in a safe environment. Our work is never done.

If you are white, don't ask your BIPOC friends to unravel all of your insecurities around the topic. Ask them to recommend books to help you better come to terms with what would be helpful. Join a group that amplifies BIPOC voices and be quiet - listening and staying in that space of mindful awareness. Challenge your thoughts when someone tells their story and you instantly think "there's no way..."

Try to remain humble and willing to learn. If you EVER think you've completely figured out how to respond perfectly to every situation, check yourself. A mark of a good practitioner is someone who is consistently learning and growing in their chosen crafts.

Taking a proactive approach to shaping your language to be more trauma sensitive will pay off in the long run. It may be uncomfortable at first, especially as you begin to realize how many colloquial phrases are rooted in some form of oppression. Recognize that your discomfort is not comparable to the discomfort you may cause someone who is struggling from being part of a group of people who face systemic discrimination.

Just trust me

Telling a client to trust you is not a great strategy. Demanding trust from a client is more likely to cause them to pull away and be leery of your work. Many people we work with have trauma that stems from a person of power betraying their trust or insisting that a person should trust them no matter what. Therefore, I don't like using phrases such as "just trust me on this."

Clients should have the opportunity to be cautious and evaluate our work for themselves. As trauma-informed herbalists, we should be accepting if someone is unsure of a natural therapy we offer. This goes back to ego: do not become frustrated if someone does not like a suggestion or is hesitant. We must be ready and willing to change paths to match whatever our clients need.

Genuine trust is built over time. Telling a client they must trust us does nothing to build that trust, and risks retraumatizing a person who has experienced previous untrustworthy experiences. Trust in a practitioner is not necessary for herbs to work. Be cautious of how you approach building trust and you will find a person begins to be more receptive to your recommendations.

Sharing your experiences

I know that sometimes we share stories of our experiences with each other in order to connect, and it can be tempting to share details of your trauma with someone who is similarly traumatized in order to show that you've also been through something difficult. This not only centers you in the conversation, it creates a situation where the person can feel triggered by hearing the details of what you've been through.

Clients may also feel you are trying to downplay their pain. Many people are told "you could have it so much worse!" and they may misinterpret your attempts at connection as an attempt to show them why it isn't so bad. Often I hear a person follow up their trauma story with something such as "but I know there are people suffering from starvation/severe neglect/insert horror story here/ so I shouldn't be complaining." The body does not discriminate: trauma responses are real even when the traumatic event didn't seem "bad" enough to cause a reaction.

Sharing your story during a client's session can also leave a person feeling unheard. The client and their needs should be the focus of the work you are doing together. There are much more effective ways to communicate that do not risk the harm that sharing trauma details can inflict.

Similarly, when you lead a group workshop, do the work to make sure you are in a space to focus on the students in the workshop. Pick a workshop topic that is something that will help people without triggering unresolved trauma of your own. If you are working to heal others, you must set yourself up for success.

I will never forget a workshop series I went to where the woman leading was still struggling with her own unresolved issues around fertility. It was a monthly women's womb-healing workshop. Each session started with a "check in" that quickly devolved into the presenter sobbing and everyone gathering around to console her... confused and uncomfortable.

I went three times before I gave up. Friends later told me this went on for the *entirety* of the nine meetings. I knew of at least two people who came away more upset about their womb related wounds than before the workshop. I suspect there were more.

I don't use this example in an effort to scare you away from helping others if you have trauma. I'm also not attempting to shame someone who is in authority showing their feelings. For goodness' sake, we are human. But a little thought into the topic and consideration around what to change after the first couple of classes went so awry could have completely changed the way this event unfolded.

"Tough love" is unnecessary pressure

Attempting to give direct orders is not beneficial when someone is already feeling overstimulated. Commands can leave a client feeling trapped and panicked. They may not feel they can handle whatever you've required of them, and they may get wrapped up in feeling inadequate or stressed around these sensations.

Offering options or inviting someone to consider a modality can be a better way to address a client who is struggling with traumatic sensations. Using phrases like "if you're comfortable, let's try a different supplement" can help them to recognize they have choices in their protocol plans.

Similarly, "tough love" is not a system I recommend if a client is struggling with trauma. Putting more pressure on someone who is already feeling like they're on the verge of breaking is likely to cause more trauma. Trauma-informed herbalists have a responsibility to respond to situations and think about their phrasing... reacting in the moment can cause someone to shut down completely and not be willing to continue on their healing journey.

I can recall a time where I was shut out due to a person not being aware of how disability could hinder a person's progress. I was attempting to explain how absolutely hopeless I felt in my practice. I tried to express how desolate I felt.

I wanted to show the counselor what wasn't working for me and why I needed specialized support. I was asking for accommodations from a wellness program I was taking. I had asked for more time on homework assignments and the counselor's body language was clear: she thought I was being ridiculous. The humiliation and shame I felt while admitting my PTSD diagnosis caused me to begin crying.

"That's too bad, I think you need to rethink your approach here. Everyone has the same twenty four hours in a day and you just need to be willing to try harder. I think that..."

My whole focus dissolved. At that moment, this person had confirmed what I most dreaded. Even though I felt like I was working as hard as I could, I just wasn't trying hard enough. I felt the heat of shame creep up my neck, realized I wasn't going to be supported, and ended the call as fast as possible - just agreeing to everything until she finally let me go.

It's been years since that conversation, and yet I've spent a lot of time thinking about that phrase. "Everyone has the same twenty four hours in a day". It sounds motivating on the surface, but it absolutely comes from a place of privilege. The tone deaf attitude of the counselor (and several other administrators in that program) was perfectly encapsulated in that one moment.

While the heat of shame was what I felt when I first heard it, I now feel the heat of anger. Anger that the person I went to for help was so dismissive. Anger that we live in a capitalist-hungry society that doesn't recognize the need to help others...

People of different socioeconomic status do not have the same twenty four hours. People with disabilities do not have the same twenty four hours. People with different social or familial support systems do not. Geographically, people may not have the same benefits.

Recognize this in your practice. One size does not fit all. The person who has to share a car with their spouse does not have the same transportation freedom that someone with their own car has. A person with chronic fatigue or long COVID may suffer for days after a mildly strenuous event. A deaf person may have to accommodate the availability of a translator (if one can even be found). A single mom with two kids does not have the same availability that a stay at home wife with no children will have.

When you notice yourself becoming tempted to react to someone's story, practice mindful awareness. In that moment, attempt to be the passive observer: only noticing the information given. Not judging. Not thinking how you would have done it differently.

Once you find yourself able to quickly access this frame of mind, you will notice it becomes easier to create protocol based on a person's individualized needs. Clients will respond favorably to being believed and respected. Your work will be more effective: you've held space for a person and not colored your recommendations with personal opinions.

Getting it right

You're not always going to get things right. We cannot plan for everyone's possible traumatic situations, but we can learn and grow as we work toward becoming more trauma-informed. Even if we lived through similar events as our clients, we may not recognize how those events affected them differently from us.

My friend Linda was in a workshop I was leading. I was attempting to quickly explain the sensation of trauma in a body and I compared it to a siren going off nonstop. In that moment, I had forgotten Linda's deep rooted fear of tornadoes and how triggering sirens could be for her.

After class, Linda discussed how she felt when this was brought up. I appreciated her willingness to share her perspective and recognized that it might be an important thing to consider in our region. We had a severe round of tornadoes tear through Alabama a decade ago. Say "April 27th" to an Alabamian and we instantly know what you mean. If I had thought about that event and its aftermath, I might have chosen a different visualization.

I apologized to Linda and validated her feelings on the matter. She was right to bring this to my attention. Even if it hadn't been something that would change the way I presented my material, I wanted her to feel heard and confident that she could bring other concerns or suggestions to me.

When someone brings a concern or mentions something you have done that triggers them, see this as a learning opportunity. Do not become offended. The temptation may be to think of yourself, "*I've done all this work - how dare they not recognize the effort I've made in becoming trauma-informed!*" Don't give in to that line of thought!

Generally people bring up a situation that makes them uncomfortable only to people they trust. Recognize that if someone is talking to you about something that made them feel vulnerable, they are doing it because they trust you to support them. Maintain an open and relaxed body language and affirm their feelings around the situation. Apologize if it is appropriate. Thank them for trusting you and bringing your attention to their concern.

Words have the power to heal and destroy

When words are chosen carefully, a trauma-informed herbalist has the ability to create a safe, healing environment for their clients. Taking time to consider different situations that face people who are struggling with trauma can help you to become a better practitioner. Making an effort to educate yourself and practice mindful awareness of your reactions to different situations can help you to change and grow into a healer that is able to help even more people.

You have the ability to start making some changes today. Come back in a few weeks, reread this chapter, notice what sticks out to you that you didn't notice before. Becoming trauma-informed is a process of shaping our minds to be more loving and supportive - even in situations we don't understand. If you haven't already, I encourage you to start that process today.

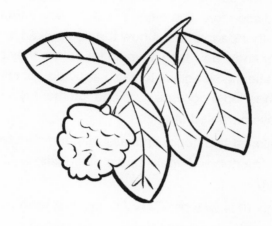

Chapter 6
Trauma Sensitive
Environments

I was struggling to breathe, dizzy, and extremely aware of how uncomfortable doctor's offices made me feel. The blaring TV and the sterile, unnecessarily bright lights were adding to my discomfort. The office manager was complaining to one of the other people about how the doctor was always late and they never knew how long it would be before they could start seeing patients. Needless to say, I struggled to stick around, but I needed a doctor's note and felt that my breathlessness warranted attention.

After almost two hours and less than ten minutes of speaking with the doctor, I finally had a diagnosis: "you've got some sort of flu."

No tests (this was pre-COVID), my final forms said the diagnosis was *actually* gastroenteritis (which didn't match my symptoms, but who was I to argue?), and he called in the equivalent of pepto bismol and a stronger tylenol dose to my pharmacy.

Did the man mix me up with someone else? Should I be concerned about how sick I feel, especially since he didn't take it seriously? Should I see someone else? Do I dare risk the struggle of dealing with another medical professional?

I left, never to go back.

Trauma sensitive spaces matter

I believe trauma sensitive environments are necessary for a person who may be struggling with trauma related stressors. It helps them to feel more comfortable in the moment, which leads to better communication with you as their herbalist. It also helps them to feel welcomed back later.

The above scenario might have gone differently if my initial hour and a half waiting on the doctor was not full of distressing environmental stimuli. The loud television, cycling through pharmaceutical commercials about high blood pressure and clots in your legs was enough to set anyone off. Add in the lighting and the unprofessional behavior of the staff... ick. I was new to the area and looking for a primary care physician: I knew that was not it.

If I hadn't been in survival mode by the time I talked to the doctor, I might have been able to articulate why I was at his facility in a more concise manner. I wondered if he may have dismissed my symptoms and wrote it off as gastroenteritis because I was so fuzzy by the time I got to him. We don't want clients leaving us and having similar doubts.

The way your office space feels to your clients can set the tone of your entire visit. Much of our work consists of having clients speak openly to us about their concerns. If your office space leaves a person feeling overwhelmed before they have even had a chance to meet you, they may not be able to articulate their needs.

When you do not convert your office into a trauma sensitive space, you risk clients not wanting to return. A unique aspect of our work is that people benefit from multiple sessions, not just one-off visits. If we make spaces that are inviting and mindfully planned, we are more likely to find clients having positive experiences and being willing to return.

When a person is struggling with trauma, their senses can become easily overwhelmed. As I mentioned in the opening of this chapter, the loud tv and bright lights caused me considerable distress. Calming music, purposeful lighting, thoughtful colors, using patterns sparingly, and remaining scent-free can help a person to feel more at home.

Instrumental music is usually considered a trauma sensitive option. As I've mentioned in chapter 5, we cannot control everyone's triggers at all times. However, instrumental music removes the possibility of words creating a triggering moment. I have several of my own recordings that I love to use as people wait. You can find many different relaxing, fully instrumental meditation recordings for purchase just by searching online.

Choosing purposeful lighting may not always be completely possible. If you're renting a space, it may come with certain fluorescent fixtures or you may find there are clauses in the lease that do not allow you to change lighting. One of my colleagues ran into this issue at her studio. She had a room she wanted to use for practitioners, but the lighting was atrocious. She got creative and placed a thin, fabric wall hanging around the ceiling fixture. Enough lighting shone through to still be functional, but the piercing brightness was muted. It was perfect!

Colors and patterns can also make a difference for someone who is struggling. My anxiety comes with a strong sense of vertigo. I despise carpets in many hotels because of this. They always seem to have funky patterns without good anchor points. If you've got chronic dizziness, you know what I mean when I say anchor points can be a survival mechanism sometimes!

Overwhelming amounts of busy patterns can create disorientation. Large chunks of neon or aggressive colors can be too much. When you're decorating your space, think of soothing tones. Do some research on which color palettes you like that are also generally accepted as appropriate for calming spaces.

Pictures and books also matter. Are you choosing a wide range of representation in your art or are you just focused on things that look like you? Does your book or magazine collection only showcase people who think like you? Is your book or magazine collection activating?

Scanning your books or magazines for possibly traumatizing subjects is an idea that I learned from my colleague Michelle Rigling, PhD. She speaks on trauma-informed herbalism through the Midsouth Women's Collective and in her work through her practice, The Cavewoman Way. She encourages practitioners to be aware of articles that may depict traumatic current events in the magazines that are delivered to your space.

I have found that Etsy is a great place for discovering art. Support a local artist if you can. One of our local yoga studio owners found some adorable prints that featured fat women in yoga poses. It was perfect for her space and made a clear statement that women of all sizes could practice without worrying about the response over their body size.

Choosing art that highlights acceptance is very personalized. I have Cherokee traditions that have been handed down from my ancestors and diluted through the lens of Appalaichan medicine. The verbal tales and legal documents passed down suggest that my ancestors were foragers and focused on gathering local herbs and vegetation. These Appalachian traditions and ancestral stories are important to me and the work I do.

Perhaps you have certain healing traditions in your ancestry that you could highlight. Perhaps there are other traditions that you feel should be represented on your walls, showing everyone who enters that healing from plants comes from many different cultures. Whatever you choose, choose from a place of love and careful understanding.

Perhaps you want to send a message of acceptance to the LGBTQ community. Perhaps you want your BIPOC clients to see themselves represented. Whatever you do, do it mindfully. If you are part of these communities then you may see inspiration amongst your peers. If you are not part of these groups, do the work and listen to their voices: we want to be appreciative of cultures without appropriating.

Similar to art, books and literature can help a person feel safe in your space. Conscientiously stocking your reference and reading corner with books that discuss different aspects of healing and herbalism can help people feel more confident in their decision to work with you.

Please recognize that there are two ways to do this: faking it or being genuine. If you choose to be performative in your space, people WILL call you out. If you pay lip service to the idea of being trauma sensitive and welcoming, people can feel it. You MUST do the work and make an effort to adapt and admit mistakes. Remember your pledge as a trauma informed herbalist: you are here to help others heal, not prove how woke you think you are.

Go fragrance free

Another easy way to adjust to being more trauma sensitive is to stop using any sort of fragrance. Scent free is absolutely the best choice in public spaces. Aromatherapy is one of my favorite modalities. I've studied clinical aromatherapy under Shanti Dechen and love utilizing essential oils in my practice. However, I do not diffuse oils in group classes or public spaces. On top of exposing people who may be sensitive, it can also trigger flashbacks.

We will talk about this further in chapter 10, but the limbic system is directly affected by scent. Essential oils can be very healing in the right context, but scents can also lead someone to a dark place in their mind. Because of how powerful scents can be, I no longer utilize them in a public space and I always tell someone what I am going to have them smell before I open an essential oil jar.

Before I studied trauma in depth, I believed there were oils that were safe to diffuse for everyone. While there were some oils that might cause sensitivity reactions, we could create a list of oils that were harmless. This was a very physically-focused system that doesn't account for emotional turmoil. Now I know better.

Even the safest oils may cause someone to remember horrible situations. My friend Rachel cannot stand the scent of lavender. She has bad memories that include lavender satchels at a relative's house. She struggles with these memories any time someone uses lavender.

Lavender! One of the most calming and beneficial options! One that we would normally have on a list of "safe for everyone" essential oils. Trauma informed herbalists MUST be aware of the power of scent.

Diffusing essential oils is only part of offering a scent free public area. Use scent free detergents for your work clothes and washable items for the workplace. Only stock scent free soaps in the bathroom. Don't wear perfume when you're going to be in your office. Work only with individual inhalation or topical application of essential oils in the office. It may seem like a small thing to you, but to someone who struggles with flashbacks at the smell of a certain detergent... being committed to a scent free environment could help them feel like they're in the right place to receive healing.

Safety

The key here is to help a person feel safe and secure in your office. They need to know that you're a person who can be trusted and that you're able to work with someone who needs specialized support. Other aspects of an office space that can help someone feel more secure include considering privacy, clearly identifying the exits, and offering gender neutral bathrooms.

We are not medical doctors and are not bound by HIPPA, but I teach all of my students that we should still recognize the need for client confidentiality. I have a release that my clients sign stating that their information can only be used in case studies or presentations if identifying information has been removed. I also do my best to not schedule friends or family to visit me directly after the end of a session. I attempt to leave a few minutes' gap so clients can leave without feeling exposed.

I love my therapist's office. It is a practice with multiple partners and they have a slightly larger space. Every time I leave, I go out one door and she goes to the other door a few minutes later to get her next patient. It's more private and allows people to flow through without interruptions.

I've seen similar set ups in several multi counselor groups. The waiting room is on one end and the person has the ability to leave out a different exit if they so choose. If you're looking for a space to expand, this could be a feature to consider.

Identifying exits so that they are easily recognizable is also important. Many building codes require this anyway, but you want to make sure clients feel they can recognize the exits. This can help someone struggling with PTSD from a violent situation, as they may feel the need to have an escape plan at all times.

Setting up your office so your client is seated in the least vulnerable spot can help as well. My therapist has a chair against one wall and I sit on a couch against the adjoining wall. This setup allows me to see the exit and there is no one between me and the exit. I don't spend time wondering how I would get out; my energy isn't tied up trying to visualize my escape route. I can focus on the task at hand: healing my brain.

Michelle Rigling, PhD, also mentions in her workshops that rearranging furniture can be disorienting to a person with unresolved trauma. Some people may find that coming into a new arrangement of furniture every few weeks is activating: now they have to find a new spot that feels safe, they have to spend energy trying to reorient to a new setup, and it may disrupt their progress that day. Consider your space and what would feel the safest, rearrange the furniture into what feels like the most trauma sensitive setup, and resist the urge to move everything once every few months.

Privacy by tinting or covering windows will also be appreciated by many clients. Some places choose to have their windows covered with specialized wraps that allow you to see out while no one can easily see inside. Window treatments can also work. Depending on your setup, you may come up with other creative ideas to help a person feel as if they have entered a practice that respects their privacy.

Single occupant bathrooms can easily be turned into gender neutral bathrooms. Cute, and sometimes sassy, signs can be found on Etsy. At one of my favorite studios in the area, the owner has put up a sign with outlines of a centaur and mermaid (in lieu of the typical man/woman outlines) that says "Whatever, just wash your hands."

Multi stall bathrooms present a trickier situation. If you are unable to designate a space for a gender neutral bathroom, brainstorm with LGBTQ+ and allies in your area to see if they have ideas you could present to your landlord. This is a tougher situation that may not have an obvious solution.

My friend Catherine directed me to the Occupational Safety and Health Administration document on gender neutral bathrooms. One recommendation in the document is to consider "multiple-occupant, gender-neutral restroom facilities with lockable, single occupant stalls". It could be possible that landlords would be willing to retrofit the bathrooms to become gender neutral with more privacy in the single occupant stalls.

If you have transgender clients, speak with them about what would help them be most comfortable. Their input can help you make the best decisions about how to adjust your space and they may have ideas you can present to your landlord. When all is said and done, creating a space that is safe and helps them feel secure is the most important thing - and to do this you <u>must</u> be willing to listen to their ideas.

Professionalism is key

Professionalism is another aspect to consider that can help a person feel safe. Holding space for a person's healing and not treating the waiting area as your own private living space can make a person feel confident they are in the right environment to be heard. I know how easily practitioners can slip into making the foyer their own hangout area, but clients walking in deserve to feel that they are centered in this space.

Highly sensitive people may notice your body language: still tense from attempting to shift out of an in depth conversation with a colleague and into holding space for your client. Instead of catching up on office gossip, spend a few minutes grounding and clearing your aura before each client. Creating a ritual that helps you to shift away from your daily concerns and into a space that puts the client first can completely shift the tone of your upcoming session.

For goodness' sake, please don't foster a culture like the doctor's office I visited. The office manager ranting about the doctor to another worker was astounding. Trauma informed herbalists should work to create a healthy office environment and hold everyone working with them to professional standards.

One of the easiest ways to create a healthy office environment is to be professional and courteous to your coworkers and colleagues. Show up on time for clients. If you have an office manager, don't run them ragged. Don't make them have to do damage control for the mistakes you've made.

The office manager at the doctor's office was clearly tired of having to ameliorate the stress from patients who had been waiting for hours to see a physician who wasn't even in the office yet. Your front facing staff can become burned out from situations they know you can control. You cannot control how others behave, but you can control how you choose to treat people you hire to help you care for your clients… and that can dictate how they act toward your clients.

Trauma sensitive as an act of service

Most of these changes are one time adjustments you can make to your clinic space. Changing lighting or color schemes to be more trauma sensitive can be as simple as repainting a wall or buying a different cover for a lamp. Finding scent free soap or changing the bathroom signs to be more inclusive are relatively simple processes. But I cannot impress upon you the difference it can make in a person's life who is struggling with trauma.

Clients come to us looking for healing, but most people initially walk into the office wanting physical relief. They may not reach out to us looking for emotional support. They may be coming in because they're finally ready to get energy back or their digestion feels off. What the trauma-informed herbalist hopes for is that when that person comes into the clinic or studio space, they find healing on all levels.

When our spaces are geared toward being trauma sensitive, we alleviate fears that we may not even be addressing in our practice. Instead of the client worrying about feeling safe or having a scent related flashback, their energy can be spent on working with us towards their healing. Instead of a LGBTQ person worrying about revealing relevant information about their gender identity or medication history, they are able to look around and see signs that we are allies, before they even meet us.

However you choose to shape your space, remember to do it from a place of service to your clients. Do not attempt to do these things in an effort to prove you're the best trauma informed herbalist in your area. Our work is effective only when we accept our place as a servant to our fellow humans. Healing on the physical, emotional, ethereal, and spiritual planes can only occur when we recognize our place as a facilitator in this experience, not the creator of the client's healing.

Now that we've addressed the space where you work, let's discuss the work of a trauma-informed herbalist. In the next chapter, I will discuss a trauma-informed herbalist's scope of practice. We will differentiate our work from that of a therapist's and discuss what to do if someone is experiencing ongoing trauma.

Chapter 7
The Herbalist's
Scope of Practice

Now you have an idea of how to recognize when someone may have experienced trauma. You know how to think about your communication and how to tailor the language you use to best support a client. You may even be able to envision what your space will look like once you have adjusted and made it more trauma-sensitive.

Now what?

What do we do when a client walks in and is clearly struggling with their trauma? How do we determine what we can do to help someone? What is a clinical herbalist's scope of practice when attempting to support someone who is still healing from traumatic experiences?

It is necessary to acknowledge that herbalists should not attempt to explore clients' dysregulation from traumatic experiences. This does not mean we do not hold powerful tools to support a person's healing journey. Our work can help a person feel more stable as they traverse the disorienting, rocky landscape of a body in a trauma response. We can hold space and allow a person to feel consistently safe and connected in our healing practice.

However, we must recognize that a trauma-informed therapist is NOT appropriately equipped to help a person explore the sensation of dysregulation; if an herbalist does this, they are outside their scope of practice. A licensed therapist can help a client work through the discomfort of being outside their window of tolerance during therapy sessions. An herbalist must resist any urge to dig into trauma processing and focus on helping a person create an energetic and physical environment in which they feel safe and secure.

Feeling safe and secure means a person benefits physiologically: their bodies will not be subjected to stress hormones as frequently. It can also cause a person to be more confident in trying new therapeutic techniques when working with their therapist. While the therapist stretches the window of tolerance through appropriate levels of discomfort and integration, the herbalist supports a client through physiological and energetic systems that passively allow the window to relax and open even further. Combine these two systems of practice (therapists and trauma informed herbalists) and clients will find themselves making leaps and bounds.

Processing trauma

You may ask, "what if a client begins discussing their trauma while they are in a session with me?" To this I say: Congrats! Your client has become comfortable or feels you are a safe place for them to open up about their struggles.

While we do not attempt to process trauma with clients, helping someone feel that they have been heard can encourage them. There are some easy techniques that can help you when a person is willing to be vulnerable and shares their experiences. Holding space for clients and allowing them to speak without our judgment or us attempting to fix their situation can create a bond of trust that allows them to feel even more confident in their healing journey.

The first thing to remember when someone opens up to you is to listen from a place of non-judgment. Your experience may be different from theirs. You may have personal ideals or beliefs that mean decisions you would have made in their situation differ from theirs. This is not the time - nor the place - to debate moralities or impose your world view onto a person.

While listening from a place of non-judgment, we should also practice active listening skills. Maintaining an open body posture, nodding or making sounds of affirmation, and acknowledging our client's feelings helps them to feel they have been heard. Creating a bond of trust through active listening allows the client to know you are an ally and you will help them get the support they need.

Expressing understanding and restating the feelings a person has communicated gives them a chance to clarify while feeling secure that you have heard them. Rephrasing concerns that they may discuss can help you when determining what herbal protocols and flower essence remedies may help them the most. Notice, we are just rephrasing what they have already told us. In a situation where someone is sharing their trauma experience, we do not want to ask questions.

Normally, one would consider asking follow up questions as a sign of being interested in the person speaking. However, asking probing questions when a trauma experience is being discussed can cause us to inadvertently activate a person's trauma response. While your client may have been in their window of tolerance when they volunteered the original information, you risk pushing them outside this comfort zone with your questions. Activating a person's trauma response while not having the tools of a therapist to help them cope can lead to retraumatization.

If a person is still in a dangerous situation, such as a domestic violence scenario, we should offer support. However, attempting to talk them into leaving could end up doing more harm than good. A person may not be ready to leave and it could cause them to close up and refuse further help. From another angle, violent abusers can escalate when a person decides to leave.

As herbalists, we are not trained to safely handle the nuance of escaping domestic violence. Always have a resource sheet with different professionals that can help clients safely plan their exit from the situation. Remind them that violence escalates and that you're concerned for their safety but also direct them to professionals who have the resources to make sure they successfully escape.

Remember: we do not need a DSM-5 diagnosis in order to determine the best support systems for our clients! Follow up questions that probe further into a person's trauma are just unnecessary for our scope of practice. Focus instead on why the client has chosen to work with you, and consider herbal protocols that support a body that has experienced trauma.

Body language

When a client initially comes to my practice, I'm going to take the time to notice their energy, body language, and other indications of where the client is at that moment. Dr. Van der Kolk has spoken about how the first two things he notices when a patient walks into his office is if they are able to make eye contact and how they are breathing. Ayurveda and other traditional healing systems suggest we should notice how loud or soft a person's voice is, whether they appear to be flushed or if the color has drained from their face, and how they move as they get settled into your space. While this can be a form of constitutional analysis, it can also help you determine how restrictive their initial protocol should be.

My students consistently hear me talk about how you cannot force someone to join you on a more intense healing journey if they are not ready to do so. For clients who are experiencing the need to heal trauma on this journey, this can become an even more important consideration. If a person is overwhelmed, you cannot expect success from recommending a protocol with so many moving pieces that it just adds to their current sensation of drowning.

As you move through a session, continue to pay attention to your client's demeanor. Take note if a person's body language shifts: becoming louder, tensing up, and their face changing color (flushing or draining) can indicate they are becoming uncomfortably close to the edge of their window of tolerance. While you cannot control their reaction, noticing if a person begins to struggle to stay regulated can help you guide your session.

If someone comes into their appointment and they are already showing signs of being highly stressed and possibly dealing with trauma, I want to approach them with a protocol that is feasible. I want them to leave our session feeling ready to succeed, not guilty or feeling incapable. Choosing the appropriate protocols is part science, part art, and part intuition.

The trauma healing process

I teach a system of determining herbal recommendations based on triangulating constitutional analysis, symptom and root cause analysis, and assessment tools that help us describe different energetic states within the body. Most people benefit from the recommendations that are derived from this system. However, for a person who is experiencing trauma related dysregulation, there is a fourth aspect that can be a game changer: where they are in the trauma healing process.

A person rarely comes to me with the intention of trying to heal from trauma. It is a secondary condition that is noted as we are working on other issues. Sometimes these other issues are directly impacted by the traumatic event, sometimes they are indirectly affected. Either way, I approach herbal protocols and natural healing modalities slightly differently for clients who are struggling with trauma.

In an ideal world, an herbalist will initially address an aspect of trauma by creating a cocoon of safety for their client. Then, once a person feels steady, they can work to build intrinsic resilience. As the person's window of tolerance expands, some of the initial "cocoon" protocols may no longer be necessary and can be removed. Once a person has worked with their therapist and feels fully integrated, they have gained lots of tools in order to naturally support them as they move forward on their healing journey.

The reality is a lot messier. I'm reminded of the memes that show a straight line, usually with a caption similar to "what success looks like". There is usually a dizzying, tangled mess of a line below this with the caption reading "what success really is". How true this is for almost any form of healing!

Building up a safety net protocol consists of finding interventions that are generally mild in nature: simple aromatherapy blends, nervine and tonic herbs, gentle lifestyle changes, restorative yoga (if it is well tolerated), and other gentle options. These are going to change from person to person.

In this initial step of working with someone who is recovering from trauma, we are going to find there is a need to create a sense of stability from extrinsic sources. Sometimes I call this my cocoon strategy (Thanks to my counselor in high school, Mrs. Ensminger, for the phrasing). Herbs that are grounding and work to activate different aspects of the nervous system are some of your best allies. Lemon balm (*Melissa officinalis*), Peppermint (*Mentha x piperita*), and Passionflower (*Passiflora incarnata* or my local favorite - *lutea*) tend to be the plants I reach for the most during initial consults. There are so many ways to approach this; we discuss herbal support more in depth starting in chapter nine.

We want clients who are struggling with trauma to have an initially positive, affirming experience. If you immediately put someone on strong herbs and begin strenuously working with energy healing or other modalities, you risk the client becoming reactivated because of overstimulation. I observed many clients leave a clinical herbalist's practice because the herbalist was too aggressive with initial protocol requirements and people were clearly overwhelmed. We must continue to meet people where they are, recognizing that sometimes it takes time to work up to stronger protocols.

Emotions and healing

Emotions and feelings can play a significant role in our protocol creations. Where a person holds stress, what they feel in moments of stress, and how they experience different emotions can help an herbalist determine which energetic formulae will best support a person. Consider these emotional contexts when you are working within your chosen traditions.

For instance, if you've been trained in Traditional Chinese Medicine, you know the system shows there are certain emotional states that point to different imbalances. Grief can manifest in the lungs. Anger in the liver.

Chakras can also give us a clue as to where imbalances may lie. I will sometimes ask a person, "when you feel <u>insert emotion here</u>, where does it manifest itself in the body?" This can frequently lead us to the throat, heart, or solar plexus chakras and my protocols will reflect that.

I may also ask about the color a person feels is associated with the emotion they have mentioned. This can help indicate chakras and give us a starting point for balancing. For instance:

"You said you have been feeling this emptiness toward your creative pursuits near your heart center. What color is it?"

"It feels orange."

Great. Now we have two chakras to work with: the heart center at the heart, and orange points us to the sacral chakra. I can make a fantastic aromatherapy blend with scents that the client likes that is also balancing to both heart and sacral chakras.

Notice how I am asking questions about the emotion, but I do not ask the person to recall the emotion in that moment. I am not a therapist, I am not here to encourage the experience and processing of these emotional states. That is something they will do with their therapist.

I use a similar technique when working with someone in guided meditations during energy healing sessions, but I slightly change the way I approach it in order to keep it as benign as possible. I will ask "where is your most obvious imbalance? What shape/color is it?" and then I ask these same questions close to the end of the session. Notice how I don't ask them to name the emotions since they are in a more meditative state.

We do not process the emotions or ask leading questions to find out more. We do not step into the realm of the therapist and begin working with someone to tackle the trauma at hand. However, we can ask what emotion a person feels, where it sits in their body, and how they would describe it.

Notice the subtle difference: asking about what is manifesting instead of asking about why the emotion is there. A trauma-informed herbalist can translate that manifestation into what energetic imbalances may exist and formulate an herbal protocol based on those imbalances. Then a person has subtle energy support that encourages the body to heal on all levels.

Clients control the pace of their healing

Sometimes people do not hold to these amazing protocols we've created and it can feel frustrating. Please always remember, traumatized people are not lazy or just refusing to do the work. On the contrary, many times people who have suffered trauma are working harder to function in basic day to day scenarios. On top of struggling with their body's reaction to trauma, many people are continuing to struggle with the systemic problems that allowed the trauma to occur in the first place. Although it is initially a paradigm shift, recognizing how others may struggle in ways that you do not will make you a stronger practitioner.

When you begin working with people from a trauma informed perspective, you enter into a position where humility and compassion open more doors than proving yourself the expert. Encouraging feedback from clients is important in establishing what parts of the protocol are working best. If someone tells you they don't have time for a certain meal plan, they don't have the energy to read a book you recommended, or they aren't ready to take the next step into a stronger herb formula, believe them. Your ability to adapt and create a flexible protocol will make you effective as a practitioner in ways that attempting to "tough love" your clients won't.

Allow clients to apply the brakes when they need to. Holistic health is not a "beam me up, Scotty" scenario. Teleportation doesn't exist in our world, this is a journey that takes time and effort. One of the best things we can do for clients is to acknowledge when they need extra time or a protocol just isn't working for them.

I would rather clients be open and honest when they feel comfortable, but that doesn't always happen. Some personality types may hesitate to tell you if they don't feel something is working. Many cultures even revere doctors and other health related professions to the point where they do not feel they have the right to question a decision made by a natural healer. Keeping notes on a person's symptom set, body language, facial coloring, vocal tone, and other observations can help you determine if something is not working as well as expected.

If you suspect a part of your protocol is not having the intended effect and a client is keeping silent about it, offer the client a choice between keeping that part or trying a substitute. This way clients can opt in for a different modality without the discomfort of telling you they are unhappy. This also keeps you from inadvertently reading a situation wrong and taking a person off a formula that is working for them.

Once an extrinsic safety net is securely in place and clients are responding well to their protocols, a trauma informed herbalist will begin to shift protocols to be a little stronger. While working to heal the physical and energetic issues a person initially came in to heal, the herbalist may also find ways to help a client build up a stockpile of natural support systems. This helps the person to become more confident and works to build an intrinsic resilience; they are able to recognize when they are struggling and which herbal interventions work best for them in that situation.

Our goal in this stage is to help a healing person begin to gain confidence in their protocol choices. We can make things even more flexible and begin to encourage exploration of different methods that might have initially been rejected out of fear. Herbal therapies that I commonly add in the second stage of healing are adaptogens. Adaptogens can help a person begin to have a stronger sense of resilience and not feel the need to stay cocooned as often. Adaptogens are literally to help the body *adapt* to stress. We will discuss the pros and cons of several adaptogens in chapter nine.

Many herbalists incorporate spiritual healing into their practices and may feel that they can start this as they move people into this second stage of healing. I am of the opinion that many healers introduce this too early in a person's healing process in an attempt to speed up the healing or help the person get a certain result sooner. Until I have been working with a client for quite awhile, I do not address the idea of journeying or guided meditations for healing. I want to be comfortable with the person being able to tell me if something is too much. I also want to be familiar with their body language and background before creating a meditation for them. We will discuss this more fully in chapter thirteen.

Stuck in survival mode

As much as I would love to sell you a story of perfect healing in all situations, not everyone makes progress into the second stage. What happens when someone is just stuck? How can we support someone who is stuck in survival mode? What do we do when they have not been able to get into a healing place?

Many people are in situations where their basic needs are not met or they are experiencing ongoing trauma and cannot bring themselves into a place to heal. This is a lot more common than many healers realize. In these cases, our recommendation needs to stay in that initial space of creating supportive protocols that evolve with the person.

I was a 911 dispatcher for almost a decade. I was a witness to many events that will haunt me for the rest of my life. I took phone calls from family, took phone calls that confirmed my worst fears, and dealt with traffic over the radio from my officers and medics that still hurts to remember.

While I studied and grew intellectually during this time, I was also facing a lot of trauma. Every time I would feel I was making progress, another wild event would occur and I would be even further in a state of exhausted shock.

It became worse when I found myself in a domestic violence situation. The ongoing stress from work and private life events took its toll. There was nothing but survival occurring during many years.

For some people, it isn't as obvious. They may be in an unstable financial situation that is leaving them worse off each month. They may not know how they will pay their bills. They may be struggling with all kinds of emotions and childhood trauma that is being reactivated from their situation.

Other people may struggle from things they don't necessarily identify as trauma. Systematic oppression of racial groups is a form of trauma, and yet many people don't realize that. They may not make the same kind of healing strides that they could make if they were not fighting against the everyday stress coming from this trauma.

How do we address this? This goes back to my comments earlier. We are on healing journeys, not teleportation events. People may be forced to meander in a situation that isn't good. When clients aren't making progress there are three things to do:

1. Believe their statements around not being able to press forward

2. Look for other options and accommodations to make your protocols more accessible
3. Have resources you can offer them

Believe your clients. Do not attempt to lecture them about why they need to do what you said. Do not argue with them about what they can and cannot handle. Don't shame them for what may appear to you to be silly choices or decisions to stay in a situation that doesn't serve them. Your job is to facilitate their situation to be as healthy as possible in their current situation.

Look for other accommodations. If something in the protocol isn't working, change it. If it is too hard for a person to remember to take an herbal formula, look for other options. Help them set alarms. If they're unhappy with the taste, change the delivery method or find a new herb. Change the time of day someone is taking the herb. There are so many ways you can adjust a client's plan to make things work for them.

Begin looking for resources now. Make connections with others in your area who offer services to people who are struggling. Keep a file on your computer with different options for counseling services, food banks, churches with social programs, whatever you run across. Not everything will be for everyone, but if you have several resources you are more likely to find someone who can help.

A note on privacy

There is no governing board in herbalism that will pull your right to practice if you are not discreet. However, this should not be taken as permission to be flippant with client information. Our clients deserve privacy and should be able to trust we are not going to air their concerns to anyone else. We talked a bit in chapter six about how to make your space more private, but there are other things we can do to protect client confidentiality.

Do not leave client intake forms lying around. Keep notes filed away and use a locking cabinet if your space is shared with others. A separate business email that uses two factor authentication keeps your clients' communication more secure.

Protect identifying information when presenting case studies or other forms of education that use client info. I change names and other information that could be used to trace my case studies back to clients. I also try to let them know if I am discussing them. My release waiver has a clause that allows me to use client information for case studies and discussions. However, I still give clients a heads up when I plan on using their progress in case studies.

Do not share information with a client's friends or family without prior written permission from the client. I also require written permission to share a client's progress with other practitioners. Sometimes this is a safety issue, like in the case of domestic abuse. This also helps to keep clients in control of their information, giving them autonomy to choose what is shared with others.

Privacy is an important aspect of being professional. To me, handling client information with care is part of an herbalist's duties. Carefully consider ways you can create a more secure practice that keeps client information confidential.

Final thoughts

Trauma sensitive herbalists do not take the place of therapists. We have very distinct, yet complementary, options that can support someone as they heal. Healers who stay in the appropriate scope of practice are less likely to cause retraumatization.

Even though most of us do not work directly with clients looking to heal trauma, many of our clients come to us with trauma as part of their etiology. If we understand where we are able to support a person struggling with trauma related concerns, we are able to confidently move forward with a plan that can help them. In the next few chapters, we will discuss plant based therapies that can be supportive of trauma related concerns.

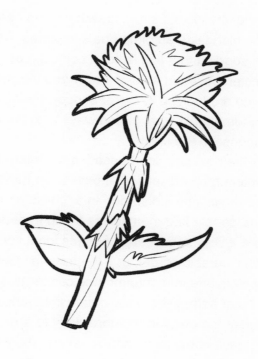

Chapter 8
The Autoimmune Connection

Many of my clients struggle with trauma based dysregulation alongside autoimmune symptoms. Research is beginning to suggest that this is not a coincidence. The dots are being connected between autoimmunity and trauma response. Herbalists who are looking to better support their clients with trauma symptoms must work to find ways to support a healthy immune response in the client.

Over the past couple of decades, a pattern has emerged. Autoimmune diseases appear to go hand in hand with post-traumatic stress disorder. In a "chicken or egg" debate, some people find themselves trying to determine whether the autoimmune disease creates ideal conditions for post traumatic stress disorder, or if the traumatic event responses precipitate into autoimmune concerns. I believe it is a combination of both: either may create imbalances in the body that cause the other to be more likely to appear. If left unchecked, these imbalances can spiral out of control into more trauma and more autoimmune disease symptoms.

Animal studies have demonstrated that gut microbiota can become significantly disrupted after trauma[1]. Dysbiosis in the gut microbiome has been linked to autoimmune disorders[2]. This combination of evidence suggests that encouraging a healthy gut flora may be one of the best ways to gently support clients who are struggling with symptoms that point toward both trauma and immune issues.

People may also be more susceptible to dysregulation following a traumatic event if their immune system is already off kilter. The Marine Resiliency Study shows that United States Marines with higher concentrations of the inflammatory marker C-reactive protein were more likely to suffer from PTSD[3]. A trauma-informed herbalist can recognize when a client may need immunomodulating herbs to support whole body healing; this whole body healing then creates a friendlier environment in which the brain can more easily heal from trauma.

Even decades after a traumatic event, the event appears to contribute to autoimmune concerns. One study showed that, compared to people who have no adverse childhood events, people with two or more adverse childhood events were 100% more likely to have a rheumatic disease as an adult[4].

The public health major in me wonders if this is due to the ongoing stress that comes with the socioeconomic struggles that can accompany a higher prevalence of adverse childhood events[5]. The chronic state of being stressed due to the injustice that many underserved communities face may play as large (or larger) a role in the creation of stress related disease in these communities... and if this is the case, as healers how can we ignore the social justice issues that plague our world?

Remember, as you are now on a journey to become a trauma-informed herbalist, you have made a pledge to recognize how others may struggle even when you do not. You've agreed that you will believe people when they say they've been hurt. You are placing yourself in a position to find ways to make proactive accommodations when possible. Shifting your mind to recognizing the ways you can support others will bring you into a place where you're a better practitioner and more effective communicator. This is how we change the world.

Immune support is one of the safest ways to start helping clients who are struggling with trauma. Immune based protocols rarely have supplements or suggestions that could retraumatize a client. Many are well tolerated and people feel much better once they begin utilizing different immune based protocols.

Nutrition

Nutrition may not be an appropriate addition to your protocols because of licensure in your state. Check your state laws to determine if you have the right to discuss nutrition with clients. Some places may allow herbalists to share education around certain diets (like the anti-inflammatory or Mediterranean diets) but may reserve the right to create personalized diet plans for licensed nutritionists or registered dieticians.

Nutrition advice is also inappropriate when a client discloses their struggle with an eating disorder. Herbalists are not trained to specifically address different eating disorders and must be willing to refer the client out to a specialist if nutritional discussion is necessary. The word "diet" might activate traumatic memories in many people, so adjust this phrasing as appropriate. Remember: our goal is to get our clients the support they need.

However, when your state laws allow and your clients could benefit from your nutritional advice, there are several options that can create good results for clients who are struggling with trauma. Clients with autoimmune concerns and trauma struggles can benefit from nutritional therapies. I'm going to start with a slightly more complex discussion around leaky gut and elimination protocols, and then we will dive into other options to help clients that need something that is less intense.

Leaky gut

Leaky gut is a theory that suggests that the reason some people struggle with excess inflammation and sensitivities is because their intestines are allowing larger molecules through into the bloodstream than they should. While there is not much research confirming this theory, it is becoming more widely accepted that intestinal permeability is a concern. Leaky gut and dysbiosis of the gut microbiota can wreak havoc on a person's immunity.

Stress can exacerbate leaky gut. A person who is struggling with unresolved trauma symptoms is likely to have more digestive and immune imbalance. Therefore, even if a person is not exhibiting symptoms of an autoimmune disorder, preventive care can stop complications from arising. We can help our clients learn about different therapeutics that could support their bodies as they continue healing.

When a client has several sensitivities to foods, that is a good indication that leaky gut is part of the concern. The most commonly blamed culprit in leaky gut cases is gluten. Many people report feeling much better after going on a gluten-free diet.

Elimination diets in general are commonly used to ameliorate the symptoms of leaky gut and they temporarily work. These elimination plans are stopgap measures that can be disheartening. What usually happens is a client will continue to have flare ups from new foods they have to eliminate or a meal that had hidden triggers. Healing must occur at a deeper level.

Restrictive diets aren't a good starting point

Highly restrictive diets have their place - once a client feels supported and safe, has a good trauma-sensitive care team, and feels ready to tackle something a bit more challenging. Eliminating triggering foods can help to speed up the healing process on an emotional and physical level. In the right context, these commonly hyped nutrition suggestions are game changers.

The problem with using elimination protocols, gluten free diets, and other restrictive measures is they assume someone has the time, energy, and financial situation to successfully implement the plan. We must always keep in mind that these more stringent protocols may be practically ineffective, emotionally disheartening, and socially restrictive. As trauma-informed practitioners, we must consider a compassionate response to the client's needs.

For many people, there may not be the time or the financial resources to implement a strict protocol. Many elimination plans can only be effective if the client cooks their own food, has access to a grocery store with specialized products, and can continue the plan for long periods of time. Socioeconomic status, family structure and dynamics, and physical health can impact a person's ability to utilize these more stringent diets.

But it doesn't end there: the emotional distress that many of our clients with trauma struggles are enduring can make these types of nutritional plans difficult. A person may be disheartened when they realize they cannot yet muster the energy to do the amount of work that goes into planning and cooking meals. Brain fog from being hyper- or hypo- aroused can make the planning even harder. Trauma-informed herbalists should be aware of this and only suggest elimination style diets if they are sure it will set the person up for success.

Nutritional restrictions commonly create unintended social restrictions. Here in the South, we gather around food. Many cultures are similar: mealtime is social time. Because of how important a person's social interactions are in their healing process, herbalists must be cognizant of this when offering nutritional protocols.

The polyvagal theory stresses the need for connection, and if nutritional changes get in the way of that connection, they can be more damaging in the long run. If we are not making mindful suggestions, we can risk creating situations for a client that can be unnecessarily strenuous… if not completely retraumatizing.

So how do we find a balance? When clients are in the early stages of healing and need strong support, how do we give them nutritional healing options that do not create the potential for more harm? Easily modifiable diets with general concepts instead of strict guidelines can help a client begin making beneficial steps toward better nutrition while not feeling restricted. Trauma-informed herbalists can start to create these accommodating protocols by familiarizing themselves with the anti-inflammatory diet and the Mediterranean diet.

Anti-inflammatory diet

The anti-inflammatory diet focuses on foods that help to reduce inflammation throughout the entire body. Dr. Andrew Weil, a pioneer in integrative medicine, frequently recommends this method as a way of eating to reduce whole body inflammation. His anti-inflammatory diet focuses on rebalancing the omega-3s and omega-6s consumed so that the body has what it needs to reduce inflammation$_6$.

This plan encourages you to eat a wide variety of fresh foods, with fruits and vegetables being a focus of each meal. Whole soy foods and cooked asian mushrooms are also encouraged. It also suggests supplements should be taken regularly to reduce nutritional gaps in the diet.

Anti-inflammatory diet education can include discussions around different types of anti-inflammatory herbs that can be used safely in culinary quantities by nearly anyone. Turmeric, ginger, cinnamon, rosemary, and sage all have anti-inflammatory qualities. Similarly to fresh foods, a wide variety of herbs will give the best result on this diet plan.

The Mediterranean diet

I've saved the best for last. The Mediterranean diet is my favorite starting place for nearly all of my clients, but I think it is particularly important for clients struggling with trauma. This nutrition plan is simple to follow, easy to adjust for different people's needs, and has flexibility that allows for a wide range of substitutions.

The Mediterranean diet focuses on vegetables, fruits, nuts, seeds, legumes, whole grains, and several different herbs used as spices. Olive oil and seafood are also staples of this rather flexible diet. It even allows poultry, eggs, and cheese to be eaten in moderation. The main things avoided are highly processed and sugary foods. The simplicity of this system means nearly anyone can find a way to make the Mediterranean diet accessible.

Herbalists should make the implementation of this diet interactive. They can encourage clients to increase vegetable intake while decreasing whole grains to create a more functionally beneficial version of the Mediterranean diet. I love working with clients to dig even further into this and find ways to "eat the rainbow."

Eating the rainbow consists of picking fruits and vegetables that are different colors. Different colors in the plants indicate different antioxidants and other beneficial constituents. The goal is to eat at least one serving of each color per week. This is an easy exercise that allows people the freedom to choose foods that work best for them.

The Mediterranean diet is also very flexible: once clients understand the basics of which foods are chosen for their nutritional value, substitutions become simple. Supplements are not needed in large amounts once a person is able to properly balance their meals. The ability to adjust this diet according to a person's needs makes it my favorite recommendation for a trauma-informed practice.

Fed is best

Sometimes nutritional support is not an option. For any number of reasons, a client may tell you that they cannot address nutritional protocols. That is ok. Trauma-informed herbalists have multiple modalities they can use to support a person.

When all is said and done, the inclusive slogan usually utilized when debating breastfeeding or formula sums it up:

"Fed is best."

Even for adults, this is true. Someone who is struggling with trauma symptoms may not be in a position to hold mental space for a perfect diet. Nonetheless: fed is best.

If a client who is struggling with trauma seems completely overwhelmed by the idea of changing their nutrition, believe them. If they appear to struggle with this in any way, that's OK. Revisit the idea later. Move ahead with less intrusive options such as nutritional supplementation, probiotics, or herbal options.

Nutritional supplementation

Nutritional supplementation can help cover gaps in someone's nutritional intake and support a healthier immune response. Someone may understand that fresh, unprocessed foods are ideal and still not be able to eat a well balanced diet. When a person is under duress, foods may not taste right or it may be a struggle to eat things they do not enjoy. That is where nutritional supplements can be beneficial.

When I work with my clients who struggle with trauma responses, we find that some of the basic nutritional supplements can quickly make a noticeable difference. If a client is on several medications, nutritional supplementation may even be safer than some of the herbal supplementation I could offer. You may find yourself commonly recommending a person supplement their diet with concentrated greens, omega-3 fatty acids, and a daily multivitamin.

Concentrated greens supplements are becoming popular. They have dehydrated greens such as kale, spinach, and broccoli. Many concentrated greens supplements will have other vegetable or grain additions for added functional nutrition benefit. Anyone will benefit from an occasional concentrated greens supplement, but this suggestion could be vital for people struggling with nutritional intake alongside unresolved trauma.

Omega-3 fatty acids are important to reduce inflammation and they help support proper brain function[7]. All of our clients need a healthy amount of omega-3s, and rarely does anyone get enough in their diet. When a client is struggling with trauma and its effects on the brain and nervous system, it becomes even more imperative that they receive this beneficial nutrient.

A daily multivitamin can help cover other gaps in a person's food intake. Many high quality multivitamins are relatively inexpensive and can help quickly make a difference. Simple changes like this make wellness feel more attainable in stressful situations.

These three things are my starting point for anyone dealing with unresolved trauma. Other supplementation is always an option. You can probably think of a whole list of things you would place in this section. As you start shifting your practice to be more trauma-informed, ask yourself: "what would be my top three essential supplements?" We will discuss even more herbs and supplements in the next chapter.

Fermentation

As we've discussed, our gut microbiota is directly affected when we are under long term stress. Clients with persistent trauma related symptoms may suffer from significant imbalances in their microbiome. This may come from stress hormones, eating habits that fluctuate alongside emotions, and other unhealthy coping mechanisms that change the gut flora. Probiotics and ferments can support a healthy microbiota as someone with unresolved trauma works to heal.

I've heard some herbalists downplay the role of probiotics and ferments in regards to trauma because they believe the answer to trauma related digestive issues is to just reduce the stress levels you are under. I completely disagree with this theory. It's privileged to think that all someone must do to be healed is recognize that stress is a problem and remove it or change the way they think about the stress. Sometimes you must replenish good bacteria in order to support a healthy nervous system in order to reduce the reaction the body is having under stress.

Fermented foods can be one of the best ways to get a wide range of beneficial bacteria into the gut. Sauerkraut, kombucha, and kimchi are common ways to introduce beneficial ferments. Sourdough is another helpful ferment that produces low gluten bread. You can buy many of these products at your local grocery store, but many people enjoy fermenting their own foods.

Sauerkraut is a cabbage fermentation. This is one of the easiest fermentations and is something I grew up watching my grandmother make. It makes a great side dish or garnish for many meals.

Kombucha is an effervescent, fermented green or black tea. Sugar is added to the tea to start the fermentation. Many people add in fruits or juice for flavor. Herbalists like to add in different medicinal and flavorful plants for added benefits.

Kimchi is a Korean vegetable ferment that is used in many soups and side dishes. It has become a popular vegetable ferment. Kimchi is seasoned with different spices such as garlic, ginger, and green onion.

Sourdough uses probiotics for a slightly different beneficial effect. The beneficial bacteria found in sourdough starter helps to break down gluten, creating a bread that is less harsh on the digestive tract. This could have a beneficial effect on immunity.

There are many other fermented foods we could discuss. Pickles, sour corn, chow chow, and fermented peaches have been part of my Southern upbringing. I encourage you to find traditional ferments that are common to your area. Look into ferments that are part of your heritage. Find different ways to connect to these nutritional supports for yourself, and then see how you could help others with similar fermentations.

Sandor Katz is an amazing fermentation revivalist who writes on ferments and does workshops all over the world. I met him at a fermentation festival and, after being completely wowed by his presentation, became totally stunned by his brain's ability to notice nuance. When I told him my full name (Lara Elizabeth), he caught that there was no "u" in Lara - just from the way I pronounced it. No one else has *ever* noticed just from conversation.

But I digress. I'm enamored with his work. His discussion around AIDS, immunity, and fermented foods is worth your time - he's careful to not suggest fermentation is a cure all, but he discusses how fermentations seem to have a place as an effective complementary strategy. His books, Wild Fermentation and The Art of Fermentation, hold prized places on my shelf. I encourage you to look into his work if fermentation fascinates you.

Probiotics

Sometimes fermented products may not be a feasible option. If a person does not have the time or the energy to keep up with the fermentation cycles, they may find themselves disheartened. Others may not have a setup to create their own ferments. The healthiest, most active fermented foods may be too expensive or not available. When this situation happens, probiotics may be the answer.

Probiotics are considered a safe option for most healthy people. There is an ongoing debate over what is considered the best therapeutic dose. The general consensus seems to currently be to find a higher-dose probiotic with multiple different strains.

I also believe in changing your probiotic supplements approximately once a month. Whenever a bottle runs out, use a different probiotic for a month. This helps to bring different strains of beneficial bacteria into the gut.

Many probiotic blends also include prebiotics. They can also be found in foods such as apples, greens, and some mushrooms. Prebiotic fibers can help feed beneficial bacteria, which in turn makes it easier for them to colonize the intestinal tract.

Rebalancing intestinal microflora is not a cure-all for immune concerns or unresolved trauma. However, this is one of the simplest ways to support clients as they continue on their journey toward healing. The mental boost that can come from a healthy gut flora could be the difference that helps your clients mov into a space of feeling safe and supported.

Leaky gut herbal support

As I mentioned earlier in the chapter, elimination diets are just a stopgap to support a person until the leaky gut is healed. There are many herbal protocols that might be helpful for someone who is struggling with a leaky gut.

White oak bark (*Quercus alba*) is a favorite of mine for addressing symptoms of leaky gut. The antiseptic and astringent properties make it wonderful for addressing unwanted bacterial overgrowth while toning the mucosal membranes. White oak bark isn't commonly touted for its abilities to help this situation, but I have found it makes a difference - especially when followed up with a strong probiotic regimen. If someone has a sensitive stomach, they may feel better taking white oak bark in a blend.

Marshmallow root (*Althaea officinalis*) is a wonderful option that also has a strong nutritional profile. Several different trace minerals and magnesium can be found in marshmallow. I love to make cold brewed tea with hibiscus and marshmallow. This preserves a lot of the mucilage and helps extract more of the beneficial nutrients of marshmallow. It's also super tasty and a favorite at my house in the summer.

Licorice root (*Glycyrrhiza glabra*) is commonly used for adrenal support, but in this instance I like it for its soothing capacity. Similar to marshmallow, its demulcent properties make it useful in gastric support teas. In some situations, small doses of licorice root can cause blood pressure issues. Usually those issues are resolved with better hydration and electrolyte balance, but clients that have this reaction should be redirected to other options.

Immunomodulatory herbs

Immunomodulatory herbs may also have a strong benefit for clients struggling with autoimmune issues and trauma. Green tea, stinging nettle, and elderberry have different, yet complementary actions that can make them helpful in this situation. You may find that adding an immunomodulatory herb to your clients' protocols helps them make more progress than just focusing on emotional support alone.

Green tea (*Camellia sinensis*) has high antioxidant levels. The polyphenols that are found in green tea have strong anti-inflammatory effects. L-theanine, an amino acid found in green tea, also has calming and relaxing effects. Green tea is an amazing option to support anyone who is struggling with a combination of autoimmune symptoms and unresolved trauma.

Stinging Nettle (*Urtica dioica*) is another herb that has a lot of beneficial nutrients and shows promise as a complementary anti-inflammatory therapy that could stabilize mast cells[8]. This may be because it is high in vitamin C, which has been shown to be useful in reducing mast cell reactions. Whatever the reason, nettle can be a good choice in certain autoimmune situations.

Elderberry (*Sambucus nigra*) has been subject to unsubstantiated rumors that it could be an immune stimulant and could potentially be dangerous for people struggling with autoimmune issues. There is no evidence that this is the case. Research seems to suggest that it is immunomodulatory and empirical evidence indicates to me that it is beneficial in many cases. The high level of antioxidants found in elderberry make it one of my favorite herbs to support people who have autoimmune concerns and trauma. Elderberry and green tea with a bit of honey is a wonderfully tasty warm beverage.

Final thoughts

Trauma-informed herbalists can recognize the need for support that digs into root causes. The immune system is one of the most important systems we can address when a person is struggling with trauma related symptoms. Research is beginning to show clear connections between immune function and severity of post traumatic stress responses.

In the next chapter, we will discuss more herbal support therapies and different body systems that could be affected. As we progress through this book, we will discuss more layers of health that herbalists may find they can support. Subtle energy, emotional, and physical aspects of a person can be affected by our work. Join me in these discussions and see ways you can support yourself, your family, and others in healing trauma.

References

1. Kelly, L. S., Apple, C. G., Gharaibeh, R., Pons, E. E., Thompson, C. W., Kannan, K. B., Darden, D. B., Efron, P. A., Thomas, R. M., & Mohr, A. M. (2021). Stress-related changes in the gut microbiome after trauma. *The journal of trauma and acute care surgery*, *91*(1), 192–199. https://doi.org/10.1097/TA.0000000000003209

2. De Luca, F., & Shoenfeld, Y. (2019). The microbiome in autoimmune diseases. *Clinical and experimental immunology*, *195*(1), 74–85. https://doi.org/10.1111/cei.13158

3. Eraly, S. A., Nievergelt, C. M., Maihofer, A. X., Barkauskas, D. A., Biswas, N., Agorastos, A., O'Connor, D. T., Baker, D. G., & Marine Resiliency Study Team (2014). Assessment of plasma C-reactive protein as a biomarker of posttraumatic stress disorder risk. *JAMA psychiatry*, *71*(4), 423–431. https://doi.org/10.1001/jamapsychiatry.2013.4374

4. Dube, S. R., Fairweather, D., Pearson, W. S., Felitti, V. J., Anda, R. F., & Croft, J. B. (2009). Cumulative childhood stress and autoimmune diseases in adults. *Psychosomatic medicine*, *71*(2), 243–250. https://doi.org/10.1097/PSY.0b013e3181907888

5. Walsh, D., McCartney, G., Smith, M., & Armour, G. (2019). Relationship between childhood socioeconomic position and adverse childhood experiences (ACEs): a systematic review. *Journal of epidemiology and community health*, *73*(12), 1087–1093. https://doi.org/10.1136/jech-2019-212738

6. Weil, A. (2017, February 6). *Influencing inflammation?* DrWeil.com. Retrieved April 1, 2022, from https://www.drweil.com/diet-nutrition/diets-weight-loss/influencing-inflammation/

7. DiNicolantonio, J. J., & O'Keefe, J. H. (2020). The Importance of Marine Omega-3s for Brain Development and the Prevention and Treatment of Behavior, Mood, and Other Brain Disorders. *Nutrients, 12*(8), 2333. https://doi.org/10.3390/nu12082333

8. Bakhshaee, M., Mohammad Pour, A. H., Esmaeili, M., Jabbari Azad, F., Alipour Talesh, G., Salehi, M., & Noorollahian Mohajer, M. (2017). Efficacy of Supportive Therapy of Allergic Rhinitis by Stinging Nettle *(Urtica dioica)* root extract: a Randomized, Double-Blind, Placebo- Controlled, Clinical Trial. *Iranian journal of pharmaceutical research : IJPR, 16*(Suppl), 112–118.

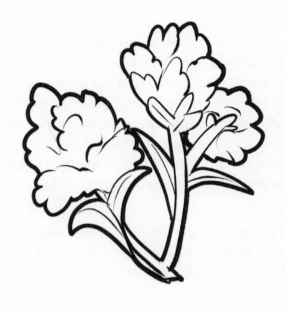

Chapter 9
Trauma Sensitive
Herbal Therapies

If you have turned directly to this chapter - bypassing our discussions around trauma and the scope of practice of an herbalist - I beg you to start over at the beginning of the book and read it through. I know the temptation to skip ahead, but this information needs to be consumed holistically the first time. Just as herbalism is an exercise of supporting the physical and intangible aspects of a person, trauma-informed work has to be considered from all angles to be truly beneficial.

Herbal therapies are amazing. That's why you're here. We love, love, LOVE our plants and the multitude of benefits that come from working with herbs.

But we also have to be mindful of how those therapies interact once someone has experienced trauma. As we discussed in the last chapter, my experience is that immune support for clients dealing with trauma tends to be a relatively benign, extremely beneficial way of working to help them heal. Everyone may react differently, but we can at least get a good feel for where we can safely start.

This chapter will dig into herbal remedies and their interaction on the nervous, endocrine, and digestive systems. We will also discuss assessment tools that require you to touch a person and concerns around herbs that could cause more stress. We will touch on herb-pharmaceutical interactions and how the different stages of healing from trauma may warrant different herbal protocols.

Flexibility is key

As a trauma informed herbalist, your goal is to create a sense of safety and security. You must always believe a person if they come to you with bizarre reactions. Clients who struggle with trauma may have unusual physical reactions due to the nervous system and endocrine system being overworked. Trying to push someone to stay on a protocol that is not working for them is uninformed, unhelpful, and potentially dangerous.

If you have a protocol that you love, begin studying how you can adjust it based on someone's needs. Start noticing other herbs that have similar actions and might fit a person better if they struggle with the original protocol. The more options you have, the better herbalist you will be.

Another thing to be sensitive to: not everyone has tons of money to throw toward a bunch of different supplements. Many people who work with us are struggling financially. Chronic illness, systemic oppression, and embarrassingly low minimum wage standards can cause people to not be able to afford fancy supplementation.

My materia medica is full of local plants, plants that I can grow myself, or plants that are relatively plentiful and inexpensive to obtain. I know the thrill of chasing an exotic plant and the excitement of working with a rare species, but the reality is we can have amazing relationships with the plants on our doorstep.

Think of dandelion. Its free spirit flows through the air, dancing. But it also grounds and runs deep, connecting us to the vibration of this planet. The versatility of this "weed" is so powerful and underutilized.

What are the local plants you can be using to support your clients? How can you help them gain access to less expensive natural modalities?

Safety and recovery

I use a few different assessment tools to determine which herbs are best for my traumatized clients. Constitutional analysis and recognizing which symptoms are trauma related help me to determine what therapies will be best. I then consider where a person is in their trauma recovery: are they trying to build safety or are they in the recovery phase?

Building safety is the main phase of trauma healing that we work with as herbalists. When people are in the early stages of learning how to heal, they need to experience safety and a supportive environment. I use a lot of nourishing herbs and gentle remedies in this phase.

The recovery phase is when a person is beginning to heal from their trauma and begins reintegrating back into their community. When a person shifts into this phase, stronger herbal formulas may be helpful. We may also find that a person is ready to try healing therapies that were too activating while they were still working to build safety.

Healing is rarely linear and a person may be in a recovery phase for awhile, but may be back in a safety phase after a jarring event. Honor what a client says they're able to handle and do not press the point if a person is traumatized and struggling. Good herbalists can shift their plan to work with anyone's needs.

Physical touch during assessment

When someone is in a session with you, do you use an assessment tool that causes you to need to touch them? Many practitioners use a form of applied kinesiology (such as muscle testing) or pulse analysis in their practice. These assessment tools can be helpful, but we also need to recognize that not everyone is going to be comfortable with being touched.

Asking a person's permission before touching them is a good start. Even better, let them "opt-in" to the experience. One of my yoga teachers, Michelle with My Vinyasa Practice, teaches the opt-in method for yoga teachers.

People sometimes feel they cannot argue with a person in authority. This feeling can be amplified in a person who is struggling with trauma related symptoms. If you ask, "can I touch you to do this assessment?" a person may agree when they aren't actually comfortable with it. It centers you and your actions, and a person may not be willing to resist and possibly create an awkward encounter.

Instead, have them opt in. Try something like this: "There is an assessment tool called applied kinesiology where I press on your hand/fingers/arm and we see if the supplement helps to strengthen you. Would you be interested in trying it?" This phrasing centers the client instead of the herbalist, allowing them to discuss their interest in the touch-based assessment tool instead of whether or not they will allow you to touch them.

In my wellness practitioner program, I work with students to learn multiple assessment tools. I encourage them to have at least three on hand, making sure they have at least one subjective and one objective method, and at least one of the methods needs to be a touch-free option. This not only makes my students strong practitioners, it creates the ability for them to be accessible no matter what a client is experiencing.

I know practitioners that work solely using applied kinesiology. Choosing this means they cannot work well with someone who is traumatized and struggles with human touch. It also means that virtual and phone appointments are ineffective. Having avenues to be able to connect even if someone physically cannot rally themselves for a visit is another way for an herbalist to be more accessible.

As we work through these recommendations, keep in mind that so much of this work is still in its infancy. We can look at the options recommended from ancient healing systems and gather some understanding. We glean more insight from the (sorely limited) published research on how herbal medicine can support people with PTSD. Conversations with other practitioners help us to gain more helpful tools. As a trauma-informed practitioner, you must continue to study and grow as this field expands.

I write this book in hopes of starting a conversation on a wider scale. Many practitioners are talking about some of the basics of trauma-informed herbal therapies, but a lot of the discussions are barely scratching the surface. I am here to encourage you to dig deeper into our work and recognize that the world has been under so much strain the past few years that we have a responsibility to take this understanding further.

This is our time. These are our people. We have to see that we can make a major difference if we begin to work to understand more about trauma. We can change people's lives if we take the time to listen, research, and learn.

I want to come back in five years and look at this book and be overwhelmed by the amount of updates I need to make. I want the second edition to become almost a rewrite... I want everyone to take ownership of the healing powers we have access to and start making changes to support their clients. We heal the world one person at a time.

Ayurveda and the polyvagal theory

In chapter three, we discussed the three states of nervous system activation that are described in the polyvagal theory. These three states, sympathetic, dorsal vagal, and ventral vagal, have similarities to the three gunas found in Ayurveda. Rajas, tamas, and sattva are the gunas, or qualities of prakriti, that determine the state of a person's mind.

Rajas is experienced in movement. It is the state of action, excitement, and stimulation. An imbalance of rajas means a person has too much energy moving throughout their body. Someone who has too much rajas in their system can show symptoms of being in a sympathetic nervous system state.

Tamas is experienced in stagnation. It is the state of slowing, inertia, and even destruction. An imbalance of tamas means someone is coming into a stagnant place where creativity and responsiveness to their environment is shutting down. A client who has too much tamas in their system can show symptoms of a dorsal vagal state.

Sattva is experienced in serenity. It closely relates to being in a ventral vagal state of calm connectedness. Sattva is not an imbalance, it is the goal state of being. It is considered the ideal state for the mind, a place of peacefulness and creation.

As with many of the discussions we are having in this book, this is a bit of an oversimplification of a nuanced system. However, I find it inspiring that the ancient wisdom found in Ayurveda has similarities to the polyvagal theory. This is more evidence we are relearning what our ancestors already knew; traditional practices have always had ways to address emotional wounds and we can learn from the systems still in practice today.

Nervous support

The nervous, endocrine, and digestive systems are important body systems that can become derailed when someone is dealing with high levels of stress. The suggestions I am making are not meant to rule your recommendations when you are helping someone struggling with trauma. They are meant to help you learn my thought process and evolve your current materia medica to support someone through your knowledge base.

Nervines, adaptogens, and herbs that support the brain are beneficial for clients who are struggling with trauma. Remember back to chapter three, where we discussed how the nervous system signals can become distorted. Herbs that support better nervous system function can help to bring things back into alignment and create more of a buffer. When there is a better buffer in the nervous system's reactions, a person may develop a larger window of tolerance and their body can focus on healing instead of straining from stress hormone overloads.

Nervines are herbs that are soothing to the nervous system. When the nervous system is hypersensitive and overreacting to stimuli, nervines can help to calm the response. This reprieve can lead to better sleep, better stress tolerance, and eventually better physical healing action.

Nervines such as skullcap (*Scutellaria lateriflora*), catnip (*Nepeta cataria*), and blue vervain (*Verbena hastata*) have calming effects with relatively few contraindications. Many nervines will work well and can be blended easily to make wonderful formulations. However, there are a couple of nervines I rarely use in initial formulae, just to exercise caution.

Valerian (*Valeriana officinalis*) is great to help with relaxation and sleep. However, it may not work well for people still struggling with traumatic effects on their body. If a person is vacillating between being hyper - and hypo- arousal, valerian may cause them to feel more alert or even jittery. Sometimes it can create a sense of more tension because of the way its energetics react with a person struggling with trauma.

Hops (*Humulus lupulus*) may also be an herb to consider cautiously as it has a tendency to damper a person's energy. If a client is struggling to come back into their body from an exacerbated dorsal vagal state, hops could aggravate this. Its hypnotic, relaxing energy may help some people but isn't my first choice for a client who is struggling to heal from trauma.

Keep in mind that each person may react differently. I have had several people find that hops and valerian worked wonders for them (especially in formulas with other nervines).

However, I've also seen clients struggle because these herbs exacerbated their feeling of disorientation. Whatever you choose for your clients, do so mindfully and with the client's best interest as your focus.

Adaptogens

Adaptogens are herbs that are known to help the body adapt to stress. Learning each adaptogen and where it is indicated can help you to determine which ones may be best for your clients. Here I will share a couple different adaptogenic plants with the thoughts I have had on them in a clinical and personal setting.

Holy basil (*Ocimum sanctum*), or Tulsi, has adaptogenic qualities that make it wonderful for someone struggling with trauma. Traditionally considered beneficial for mental acuity and concentration, I like to reach for holy basil when someone is dealing with a feeling of brain fog. With no known contraindications, it is commonly well tolerated.

Ashwagandha (*Withania somnifera*) has great anti-inflammatory properties on top of being a wonderful adaptogen. When I have a client who is struggling with other inflammation related symptoms on top of their trauma, I encourage them to try ashwagandha. Because of its popularity, ashwagandha has become easy to find. Be aware that some supplements will market ashwagandha in capsules but when you read the label it is blended with other adaptogens.

Shatavari (*Asparagus racemosus*) is my favorite adaptogen for people who have been in a traumatic situation for so long that they feel they have nothing left. It has a very nourishing feel that creates a sense of hope. In moments of complete exhaustion, I reach for shatavari and she reaches back. That feeling of connection is irreplaceable.

Adaptogens have become overused and aren't the catch-all remedies for energy and stress that some people make them out to be. They are wonderful herbs, but abusing them to gain a bit of short term energy is not going to allow a person to heal properly. I always utilize adaptogens alongside other herbs that can support the nervous system's rebalancing.

Rhodiola (*Rhodiola rosea*) is the one adaptogen I don't use at first with clients who have unresolved trauma. It's generally a good adaptogen for anyone who needs a post-workout pick me up or endurance support. However, in a client who is struggling with trauma, rhodiola can create a jittery sense of anxiety, especially when someone is prone to a hyperarousal response. Therefore I usually start someone elsewhere, then we discuss rhodiola as they progress into their recovery phase.

Sleep

Sleep can easily be disrupted when someone is dealing with a trauma response. Low quality sleep can exacerbate a person's trauma related symptoms and even cause new ones to occur. If someone is struggling with sleep and they have unresolved trauma, there are a few things we can do to help restore quality rest as they work to heal.

Sometimes hyperarousal can disrupt sleep patterns. When a client comes in and states they are only sleeping a couple of hours a night and they're exhausted, I am not surprised. That is a common symptom of hyperarousal.

However, If a client comes in and tells me they are consistently wired after sleeping only a couple of hours a night, I encourage them to mention this pattern to their therapist. It could be a sign of other mental health concerns. Encouraging your clients to self advocate can help them get support that they need - no matter what the underlying cause.

Before I ever touch any herb recommendations with a client, we discuss sleep hygiene. Having a regular routine that encourages the body to relax and prepare for a good night's sleep can make a difference. Subtle changes such as consistent sleep times, caffeine intake, pre-bedtime activities, and limiting screen time can significantly improve sleep quality. These things seem silly at first, but my clients who are able to consistently implement sleep hygiene practices have an easier time reclaiming their sleep.

Going to sleep and waking up at the same time every day can help the body get into a rhythm. Even if sleep is elusive at first, getting up at the same time every day can help a person reset their biological clock. Starting this habit will help the body be more prepared to accept sleep at the right time.

There are several reasons as to why limiting caffeine intake can be important for healing. Limiting oneself to small amounts of caffeine first thing in the morning is the most common recommendation I make. Everyone's sleep quality is affected when they drink caffeine, whether they realize it or not. For someone who is struggling to get good sleep, limiting or eliminating caffeine intake can make a world of difference.

Having a pre-bedtime routine that stays relatively consistent can help signal to your body that it is time to go to sleep. I tend to encourage clients to add one thing at a time instead of trying to completely revamp their habits. Drinking a cup of tea, listening to calming music, meditating, journaling, or reading a few pages in a book may be things you consider adding to your pre-bedtime routine.

Pre-bedtime routines can include lowering the lights to help the body prepare for sleep. Limiting screen time in the evening aids in melatonin production. For some people who struggle with overstimulation, blue blocker glasses throughout the day or starting in the afternoon may be warranted.

Relaxing herbs such as lavender (*Lavandula angustifolia*), chamomile (*Matricaria recutita*), and lemongrass (*Cymbopogon citratus*) can be great herbs to use in a tea near bedtime. The stronger nervines we discussed earlier in this chapter can also be helpful. Herbs such as valerian and hops are also useful.

"But, Elizabeth, you just said to be careful with valerian and hops?"

Yes, I did. All of these herbs can be helpful when utilized appropriately. Just keep the situations I am describing in mind and proceed with caution. Just as certain herbs work better with certain constitutions, certain herbs work better with certain nervous system states.

A final note on melatonin: it is overused. Most people need very little, if any. When clients come to me and tell me that they have nightmares or their insomnia is worse after melatonin, I usually find that they were taking very large doses.

For reference, I only take melatonin on nights that I am not tired at all. I keep the dissolvable tablets and use ⅓ of a tablet when necessary. This means I'm taking a little over 1 mg per dose… and my doctor has even said he thinks I wouldn't need that much to get quality sleep.

High quality sleep means the body is able to create an environment where healing is more likely to occur. Someone who is struggling with sleep may have higher inflammation levels[1]. As we touched on in the previous chapter, reducing inflammation can help to make it easier to heal trauma.

Anti-inflammatory support

We've discussed some lifestyle changes that can support anti-inflammatory actions in the body. We've also touched on nutritional changes that can create an anti-inflammatory response. Anti-inflammatory herbs can be an amazing complement to these other shifts. I love using plants that have anti-inflammatory properties and are also beneficial to the nervous system.

Gotu kola (*Centella asiatica*) has a calming effect on the nervous system and a general tonic action on the body. I love gotu kola because it exhibits some cardiovascular support on top of its anti-inflammatory properties[2]. Gotu kola is best used in short spurts, taking it for a few weeks and then coming back to it later.

Green tea (*Camellia sinensis*) is an option that I recommend as an everyday hot infusion for many of my clients. As I mentioned in the last chapter, green tea is a great immunomodulatory option. L-theanine, a component of green tea, has beens studied for its ability to reduce PTSD-like symptoms[3]. If someone is prone to hyperarousal, I will recommend only drinking the tea in the morning because of its caffeine content. Generally, green tea is well tolerated in moderate amounts.

Turmeric (*Curcuma longa*) is another anti-inflammatory herb that is helpful for many people struggling with trauma. One animal study suggested that turmeric may be helpful in attenuating PTSD symptoms[4]. Unless your focus is on reducing inflammation in the colon, you will want to add some black pepper (*Piper nigrum*) for better absorption.

Endocrine support

When a person is stuck in a state of fight or flight response, their endocrine system can be pushed into overdrive. The adaptogens discussed earlier in this chapter will also have beneficial impacts on the glandular system. Remember, adaptogens help the body adapt to stress. This dual endocrine/nervous system support action makes adaptogens a great option when you're trying to keep a protocol within a certain budget.

Supporting the thyroid, pancreas, and adrenals during high stress situations can help a person avoid further health frustrations. The cortisol that is released by your adrenals can directly impact the function of other glands. Chronically elevated cortisol levels can create a situation in which glucose is continuously produced, creating insulin resistance and straining the pancreas. This can lead to weight gain, cardiovascular struggles, and eventually metabolic syndrome.

Barberry (*Berberis vulgaris*) is a plant that has a high level of berberine. Berberine is becoming known for its ability to fight insulin resistance, obesity, and metabolic syndrome[5]. It is showing a lot of promise in supporting healthy glucose levels. Other plants, such as Oregon grape (*Mahonia aquifolium*) also have lots of berberine.

Ginger (*Zingiber officinale*) is a culinary herb with many touted benefits. Recent studies are beginning to look at how ginger may reduce blood sugar levels[6]. Its spicy root also has a warming and grounding affect.

Milk thistle (*Silybum marianum*) has been traditionally used as a liver support herb. More studies are being done that show its hepatoprotective mechanisms[7]. While not directly acting on the pancreas, it appears to have a slight effect on insulin resistance.

Digestive support

As we discussed in the last chapter, the digestive system plays a strong role for health in general - but even more so for someone struggling with trauma. Herbal digestive system support will depend on the symptoms a person is experiencing. One category of herbs that can strongly benefit the digestive tract are bitters.

Bitters help to stimulate digestion and can be particularly useful if someone finds they are struggling to eat because of stress. After my dog passed, I found that digestive bitters were helpful when I needed to eat but had no appetite. Ginger and milk thistle could be considered digestive bitters. Dandelion and alfalfa are two nutritive bitters I find helpful for clients needing digestive support.

Dandelion (*Taraxacum officinale*) has lots of beneficial properties and the plant can be prepared in many different ways. The root is traditionally seen as a digestive bitter, but almost all parts of the plant can be beneficial. The baby leaves in the spring are nice on a salad. The root can be roasted and makes an interesting addition to many brewed drinks. Dandelion flower cookies and dandelion jelly are surprisingly tasty.

Alfalfa (*Medicago sativa*) is a bitter that has many trace minerals. We see alfalfa used in many healing traditions across the globe. Alfalfa can cause lupus flare ups, so I avoid it when I am working with a client who has lupus or an autoimmune issue that is yet to be diagnosed.

Herb - pharmaceutical interactions

There are some concerns that an herbalist should carefully consider when working with someone who has a background of trauma. Many clients will be on some form of SSRIs or other psychotropic medication. These pharmaceuticals can have interactions with several herbs.

If someone who is actively struggling with trauma is working with me and I suggest an herb that could have interactions, I go ahead and tell them about the interaction. Even though they may not currently be on anything, I want them to know they should stop it if their psychiatrist puts them on a medication that could interact.

Drugs.com can be a useful source for commonly reported interactions. Keep in mind that every single known interaction is mentioned on the site, some of which don't have clinical significance. However, it is a great resource if you have a client who is taking a medication with which you are unfamiliar.

Pay attention to unique mental health-related herbal concerns

Another concern is something that I have noticed as I have begun working with more people who are presenting with trauma symptoms. Herbs that have a sensation of untethering a person from this physical form can be difficult to work with at first. Recommend these carefully, recognizing how a person could feel more dissociated after their use.

If a person is in the early stages of healing from trauma, they may struggle with feeling connected and present. Gaslighting may have caused them to become disoriented and they may struggle to find a way afterward to set themselves upright. The sensations coursing through the nervous system can also be disorienting. Sometimes these sensations can be exacerbated by herbs that can leave us with a "floaty" feeling.

I have had several practitioners report to me that Damiana (*Turnera diffusa*) leaves their clients with trauma feeling a bit unnerved from the out of body sensation it can cause. This generally safe herb can all of a sudden feel unsafe for someone whose trauma response is to go into a dorsal vagal state. I avoid use until a person is feeling more grounded and ready for its effects.

St John's wort (*Hypericum perforatum*) is another herb that must be considered carefully with clients struggling with trauma. It was touted in the late 90s and early aughts as a miracle herb for depression. Since then, we've learned that it has its drawbacks.

I found out about St. John's wort's ability to mess with the mind from personal experience. I was at a magnet high school and had become depressed. I began taking (probably too much) St. John's wort in order to combat it. I then began having auditory hallucinations.

I am lucky, when I stopped taking St John's wort the hallucinations stopped. Since then, multiple case reports have come out detailing the possibility of psychosis-like symptoms[8,9]. Therefore, I do not ever recommend St. John's wort internally for a person who is struggling with unresolved trauma.

Trauma-informed delivery methods

How we choose to offer herbal remedies can also come into play in trauma-informed care. Clients may struggle with swallowing large capsules or they may not be able to drink alcohol. Taking an herbal medicine making course (like the one offered by Sam Coffman and Suchil Coffman-Guerra through their school, Herbal Medics Academy) can help you to be prepared to pivot your recommendations as necessary.

For instance, if someone struggles with alcohol or has a religious objection to alcoholic preparations, I do not offer tinctures. Instead, I turn to glycerites for any liquid preparations.

Glycerties are herbal extractions done in a combination of glycerin (the sweet part of fat) and water.

Quick adjustments like this can make a session go more smoothly. Clients will appreciate the lack of struggle you put them through. When we proactively notice how we can accommodate different people's needs, we are practicing trauma-informed care.

We need more herbalists to pay attention

This just scratches the surface of how we can adjust our plant medicine to help others. We need more information about how people respond to herbal treatment after trauma. I encourage you to observe, notice what is working, and communicate with other practitioners. If we can talk to each other, we will start to get a better picture of what is happening and what works best for different scenarios.

That's my dream: discussions around the feasibility and effectiveness of herbal based therapies for people struggling with trauma symptoms. Research that leads to evidence-based herbal medicine that shows how this works best. In the meantime, as trauma-informed herbalists, let's work to learn more so our clients can have better outcomes.

Over the next few chapters, we continue our discussion in plant medicine. I encourage you to find different applications that inspire you to dig further. If you're already well versed in these modalities, look at the way I adjust them to be more trauma-informed. Use these ideas as a jumping off point for better care for your clients, your family, and yourself.

References

1. Irwin, M. R., Olmstead, R., & Carroll, J. E. (2016). Sleep Disturbance, Sleep Duration, and Inflammation: A Systematic Review and Meta-Analysis of Cohort Studies and Experimental Sleep Deprivation. *Biological psychiatry, 80*(1), 40–52. https://doi.org/10.1016/j.biopsych.2015.05.014

2. Razali, N., Ng, C. T., & Fong, L. Y. (2019). Cardiovascular Protective Effects of Centella asiatica and Its Triterpenes: A Review. *Planta medica, 85*(16), 1203–1215. https://doi.org/10.1055/a-1008-6138

3. Ceremuga, T. E., Martinson, S., Washington, J., Revels, R., Wojcicki, J., Crawford, D., Edwards, R., Kemper, J. L., Townsend, W. L., Herron, G. M., Ceremuga, G. A., Padron, G., & Bentley, M. (2014). Effects of L-theanine on posttraumatic stress disorder induced changes in rat brain gene expression. *TheScientificWorldJournal, 2014*, 419032. https://doi.org/10.1155/2014/419032

4. Lee, B., & Lee, H. (2018). Systemic Administration of Curcumin Affect Anxiety-Related Behaviors in a Rat Model of Posttraumatic Stress Disorder via Activation of Serotonergic Systems. *Evidence-based complementary and alternative medicine : eCAM, 2018*, 9041309. https://doi.org/10.1155/2018/9041309

5. Firouzi, S., Malekahmadi, M., Ghayour-Mobarhan, M., Ferns, G., & Rahimi, H. R. (2018). Barberry in the treatment of obesity and metabolic syndrome: possible mechanisms of action. *Diabetes, metabolic syndrome and obesity : targets and therapy, 11*, 699–705. https://doi.org/10.2147/DMSO.S181572

6. Nam, Y. H., Hong, B. N., Rodriguez, I., Park, M. S., Jeong, S. Y., Lee, Y. G., Shim, J. H., Yasmin, T., Kim, N. W., Koo, Y. T., Lee, S. H., Paik, D. H., Jeong, Y. J., Jeon, H., Kang, S. C., Baek, N. I., & Kang, T. H. (2020). Steamed Ginger May Enhance Insulin Secretion through KATP Channel Closure in Pancreatic β-Cells Potentially by Increasing 1-Dehydro-6-Gingerdione Content. *Nutrients, 12*(2), 324. https://doi.org/10.3390/nu12020324

7. Doostkam, A., Fathalipour, M., Anbardar, M. H., Purkhosrow, A., & Mirkhani, H. (2022). Therapeutic Effects of Milk Thistle (*Silybum marianum* L.) and Artichoke (*Cynara scolymus* L.) on Nonalcoholic Fatty Liver Disease in Type 2 Diabetic Rats. *Canadian journal of gastroenterology & hepatology, 2022*, 2868904. https://doi.org/10.1155/2022/2868904

8. Ferrara, M., Mungai, F., & Starace, F. (2017). St John's wort (Hypericum perforatum)-induced psychosis: a case report. *Journal of medical case reports, 11*(1), 137. https://doi.org/10.1186/s13256-017-1302-7

9. Joshi, K. G., & Faubion, M. D. (2005). Mania and Psychosis Associated with St. John's Wort and Ginseng. *Psychiatry (Edgmont (Pa. : Township))*, 2(9), 56–61.

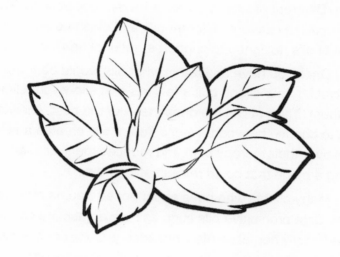

Chapter 10
Aromatherapy

Aromatherapy has a strong beneficial effect on our emotional state when appropriately utilized. When inhaled, the molecules of different essential oils cause reactions in the limbic system. Different oils have different therapeutic actions. This chapter outlines several different oils and digs into an energetic system of oils designed to support emotional healing.

Once you have an idea of what oils would be most beneficial for your client, pull a few oils and allow your clients to smell them. Then utilize the ones they like the best. Allowing clients to choose between a few different oils creates a sense of control over their therapy plan and reduces the likelihood of creating a blend that could retraumatize them.

Many clients who have experienced trauma may be on a budget. Cost prohibitive oils such as rose or jasmine should be required only when absolutely necessary. Consider finding other, less expensive oils that have similar therapeutic properties to have on hand. Rarely do I find I have to utilize an expensive oil anymore.

Below is a list of oils I use frequently for emotional healing. I also outline some of the more costly oils that can be replaced with less expensive options. Then we discuss the system I use to blend essential oils to mend multiple chakra imbalances.

Essential oils for emotional healing

Here are several essential oils that have emotional healing properties and are usually reasonably priced for anyone's use. I chose over twenty inexpensive oils that I have seen clients benefit from when dealing with trauma. This list is not exhaustive; there are several other oils that could show benefits for people who are working to heal from traumatic experiences.

Sweet Basil (*Ocimum basilicum*) is fantastic for someone struggling with head and body aches stemming from holding tension. It has a wonderful tonic action when a person is feeling frayed around the edges. I like to combine it with sweet orange and lavender to help occasionally restless sleep.

Bergamot (*Citrus aurantium spp. bergamia*) supports the body by helping a person let go of anger. This balances emotional energy held in the liver and helps to bring nervous digestion back into alignment. I love using this to bring uplifting energy to a blend when someone is feeling brain fog from exhaustion. Blend with black pepper when a person describes frequently feeling disconnected and fuzzy.

Black Pepper (*Piper nigrum*) has the handy ability to support a person who is dealing with a lot of nerve related pain. It is known for being a clarifying oil and can cut through the mental fog that comes from emotional upheaval. I frequently use it for appetite related emotional support. For instance, it can help encourage a healthy appetite when someone is struggling with nervous related weight loss. However, black pepper can also help reduce cravings in a person who is eating out of nervousness.

Cedarwood Atlas (*Cedrus atlantica*) is loved for its ability to help people reconnect to themselves. It has a grounding effect that works well on people who feel disconnected to their true purpose. However, because of overharvesting and sustainability concerns, I tend to more frequently turn to its distant cousin, virginiana.

Cedarwood Virginiana (*Juniperus virginiana*) has a slightly more biting undertone. It has similar emotional healing qualities as Atlas, and is considered more sustainable. It helps people feel more centered and able to make better decisions when under stress. Virginiana is stronger than Atlas, so utilize Atlas for children and people who are more sensitive.

Cinnamon Leaf (*Cinnamomum zeylanicum*) is my go to when someone feels listless and weak from struggling. It can add a sense of protection and energetic support. I like to blend with fruity or other spicy scents to help people feel comforted. Great when someone who has been through a traumatic event has a general sense of malaise.

Cypress (*Cupressus sempervirens*) is a phenomenal companion oil for someone who is in the midst of a transition. This is a fantastic oil to incorporate when a person is shifting away from a long term traumatic situation and into a healthier space. Self-forgiveness is unlocked with the use of cypress. The transformational qualities can also help someone who is grieving to move forward into their new reality.

Eucalyptus Globulus (*Eucalyptus globulus*) encourages a sense of adaptability and resilience. It can help to jumpstart the emotional healing process. I like to include eucalyptus when someone is struggling to release the feeling that their trauma is part of their identity. Instead of a person strongly holding on to their struggles, they are able to acknowledge the trauma's place as part of their past and begin looking toward a healthier future.

Fennel (*Foeniculum vulgare*) is a balancing oil for almost any constitution. I love to blend it with orange and peppermint to relax nervous digestion issues. Also wonderful for releasing the type of energetic blockages that create a sense of brain fog. Its detoxifying effects seem to help my clients release toxic situations and people from their lives.

Frankincense (*Boswellia serrata*) has grounding and protective qualities that make it great for nearly any sort of stress. It also has spiritual connotations that mean it is useful when someone is working to get realigned with their higher purpose. Because of overharvesting concerns, I rarely use frankincense. We will discuss a flower essence substitution for higher purpose connection, wild oat flower essence, in the next chapter.

Geranium (*Pelargonium graveolens*) is a relaxing oil that I find helpful in sleepy time blends. It can also help a person who is feeling jumpy, as if they're living in a horror movie and a jump scare is just around the corner. Geranium can be a great companion when a person needs a clear head walking into a stressful situation.

Ginger (*Zingiber officinale*) has an earthy, woody feel that adds a sense of grounding and adrenal support. When someone is struggling with energy dips throughout the day, ginger can help to create a more steady sense of energy in their body. It can support the circulatory and digestive systems when they are easily affected by stress.

Lavandin (*Lavandula hybrida*) is a hybrid lavender made from *angustifolia* and *latifolia*. It has a sharper, more camphorous smell. It creates a feeling of support and an emotional buffer for people who are trying to recuperate. Lavandin pairs wonderfully with sweet basil for those struggling with frayed nerves.

Lavender (*Lavandula angustifolia*) is the sweeter half-sister to lavandin. While lavandin creates a sense of support, lavender allows a person to completely relax. It is a wonderful tonic for a person who has been overthinking situations. I find lavender helpful for situations where a person is needing to feel a sense of relaxation - even when the storm rages around them.

Lemon (*Citrus x limon*) has an energizing scent and is able to support healthy immune function that may be lacking in times of extreme stress. It is my "summer oil" that brings a feel of light and vitality even in the dead of winter when many people struggle. I like to blend this with ylang-ylang for a great catch-all for stress related bouts of low energy.

Palmarosa (*Cymbopogon martinii*) has cooling and replenishing properties. It helps when someone is trying to recuperate from habitual burnout. While it won't make much of a difference if the person continues to work themselves into the ground, it can work wonders when the person chooses to rest. It easily cuts through clouds of brain fog to bring in a feeling of light. When combined with lemon and thyme, palmarosa makes a great blend for relieving fatigue.

Patchouli (*Pogostemon cablin*) is an amazing grounding oil that supports the root chakra. When I have clients that have symptoms reminiscent of adrenal fatigue, I like to use patchouli. Feeling wide awake at night and then feeling exhausted throughout the day? Blend it with lavender and bergamot and use in the early afternoon to help reset your system.

Peppermint (*Mentha x piperita*) is another phenomenal option for digestion issues that are related to stress. I also love to utilize peppermint when someone is feeling angry after a traumatic episode. It helps to redirect this energy into a healthier path. Peppermint is especially helpful if the anger is creating dizziness or headache from tension.

Rosemary (*Salvia rosmarinus*) is perfect for someone who is losing short term memory because they are struggling from trauma. My grandmother always says "rosemary for memory." This seems true of both the herb and the essential oil. Use it first thing in the morning to shift out of the dream world and into a state of alertness.

Sage (*Salvia officinalis*) is wonderful to help create the feeling that all is well. It has a warming effect that brings renewal to a person who is grieving. It has a relaxing effect on muscles that have become achy from tension. Blend with lemon for someone who is struggling to cut through the fog of stress-induced exhaustion.

Spearmint (*Mentha spicata*) is the gentler half sister to peppermint. Great for people who are generally more sensitive. It has similar therapeutic properties to peppermint, with a gentler cooling energy. It is fantastic in a blend with sweet orange and lavender for relaxation effects that can be utilized anytime of the day.

Star Anise (*Illicium verum*) helps when someone is struggling with trusting their intuition and it is causing them to be bristly toward others. People may struggle to trust their connection with others after a trauma, especially if it was perpetrated by a close friend or relative. Blend with sweet orange for someone who finds themselves responding poorly in social situations.

Sweet Orange (*Citrus sinensis*) uplifts and energizes while releasing nervous tension. Its harmonious energies allow for a balancing effect on a person who has been struggling with unresolved trauma. Great for caregivers who are dealing with burnout. Add sweet orange to almost any blend and your clients will reap benefits from it.

Ylang Ylang (*Cananga odorata*) is a favorite of mine because it has such a balancing effect on the emotions. When someone is feeling jittery, it can help them to relax. When someone is feeling fuzzy or flat, it can help brighten their mood. Confession time: I use 3rd degree ylang ylang, which is the 'weakest' of the three options, but it still gets phenomenal results.

Cost prohibitive oils

Some oils have wonderful beneficial properties, but their extraction processes are difficult and cause them to be extremely expensive. These cost prohibitive oils are ones that I do not regularly use with clients. I have worked to find other oils that I can use in their place. I encourage you to find oils that have similar energetics and therapeutic properties for you to use with clients.

If you choose to utilize these oils, make sure you're getting them from reputable sources. All oils need to come from a good source, but highly expensive oils are even more likely to be adulterated with less expensive oils or carrier oils. For instance, melissa is sometimes cut with lemongrass and citronella oils in order to create a similar scent for less.

Rose (*Rosa centifolia*) has a sweet, floral scent that creates a sense of encouragement and hope. When the nervous system is creating imbalance in the circulatory system, rose can be a good tonic. While it is difficult to replicate the energetic and therapeutic actions with a single oil, I have found a combination of lavender and geranium can create a similar feel.

Helichrysum (*Helichrysum italicum*) is an oil that many practitioners reach for when a person is struggling with adrenal fatigue or exhaustion. Helichrysum is especially helpful as a person is getting out of a bad situation; It helps a person be more forgiving toward themselves. Cypress or ginger can have similar energetic effects.

Jasmine (*Jasminum grandiflorum*) is by far one of my favorite plants, even though its essential oil is cost prohibitive in practice. Its balancing effect makes it a great catch all, especially if someone is struggling with symptoms that seem to vacillate from too much energy to too little. Ylang ylang has a similar action and is my go-to substitution for jasmine.

Melissa (*Melissa officinalis*), also called lemon balm, has a gentle lifting action that can be helpful in times when someone is feeling low. If someone has twitching in muscles that occurs when they are stressed, I include lemon balm in their blend. I hate that it is so expensive to get the essential oil, but lemon balm grows so abundantly in our area that I tend to use the whole plant for emotional healing and get similar benefits.

Myrrh (*Commiphora myrrha*) is great when a person is overthinking situations and "chewing the cud" over their experiences to the point where it is a detriment to their well being. Myrrh also helps these type A people with relaxation and connecting to a higher purpose. Lavender and fennel are good substitutes, depending on the person and the type of situations on which they tend to ruminate.

Neroli (*Citrus aurantium*) is an oil that means springtime and carefree happiness to me. One of my favorite songs ("Orange Blossoms" by Mofro) plays in my head as I think of this oil. This upbeat scent cuts through the cloudiest moments and creates a sense of hope. Sweet orange works just as well many times, even though it has a completely different scent profile. The similar energetics allow it to be a useful substitute. Palmarosa is another energetically similar oil with a more floral scent.

Vetiver (*Chrysopogon vetiveria*) has digestive and nervous system balancing benefits that make it a wonderful addition to many blends. It helps a person release frustration and become focused on their healing. Peppermint and ginger have similar benefits at a fraction of the cost, making them my go-to replacements.

Aromatherapy and chakras

One way I love to use essential oils is to balance the chakras. Because the seven main chakras have such clear emotional components, I began to use my aromatherapy-based emotional healing techniques to support the chakra system. This system has been an amazing help for many of my clients. It is easy to implement, creates amazing blends, and has a lot of useful applications.

The seven main chakras that are found along the midline of the body have direct effects on the nerve plexuses found in their corresponding locations. Many teachers theorize that the chakras are the link between our etheric bodies and the proprioceptive system. When chakras are out of balance, the body may register an imbalanced response to external stimuli, exacerbating trauma related symptoms.

Chakras are much more nuanced and powerful than I have space to describe in this chapter. The following information is a brief overview in order to help you visualize how I utilize aromatherapy to balance the chakras for different emotional concerns. I will go more in depth into the chakras and trauma in chapter fifteen.

This system implements seven scent families: one for each of the chakras. Several oils can fall into each of the scent categories, meaning you are likely to find at least a few oils that match the chakra that needs balancing. Some oils may even be classified into more than one scent category. Many of the scent families blend well with each other, making it easy to balance multiple chakras with one blend.

The root chakra, muladhara, is located at the base of the spine. It is associated with the adrenal glands. A healthy root chakra can help a person feel grounded and centered. It is the energetic hub that helps our creative thoughts become physical reality.

When someone is struggling with unresolved trauma, the root chakra may be weakened. This may cause a feeling of being untethered. A person may find themselves struggling to sleep at night and then being exhausted and barely able to function the next day.

Earthy scents, such as patchouli or carrot seed, can help to bring balance to the root chakra. These scents are reminiscent of being connected with the earth; grounding into the soil and rooting oneself in communion with the resonance of our planet. Earthy scents blend well with woody and minty scents.

The sacral chakra, svadhisthana, is located near the navel. It is associated with sexuality and creativity. If someone begins feeling unable to create or loses their inspiration, I always look to see how I can support their sacral chakra. Think writer's block: that's almost always a sacral chakra imbalance.

When someone has gone through a traumatic event, it is common for them to lose interest in creative passions. Assuming the trauma was unrelated to their creative pursuits, one way to help the healing process is to resume creating. Whether their interests lie in making music, painting, acting, or whatever else, creativity can heal. It may feel stilted at first, but nourishing a traumatized person's sacral chakra can help to make these activities naturally flow.

I associate the sacral chakra with herbaceous herbs. Think kitchen spices such as rosemary, sage, and oregano. These are usually deeper scents with a hint of warmth that can help stir ideas into a creative space. Herbaceous scents blend well with woody and minty scents. Many also pair well with citrus.

The solar plexus chakra, manipura, is located in the upper abdomen near the solar plexus. It is associated with the pancreas, or more specifically the islets of Langerhans. These cells secrete insulin and glucagon in response to blood glucose levels. It is also the energetic area that dominates a person's sense of self.

When a person experiences trauma, stress hormones are released into the bloodstream. These hormones can cause blood sugar levels to be erratic. Long term stress can cause more issues that stem from changes in blood sugar. Supporting the physical body is important, but adding a complementary approach of supporting the solar plexus chakra may also help.

Trauma also can cause a person to struggle with their sense of self. Experiencing gaslighting or suffering from survivor's guilt may cause a person to second guess their decisions. Self confidence may plummet. Energetically nourishing the solar plexus chakra can help a person challenge negative self talk that stems from traumatic experiences.

The solar plexus is connected with woody scents. Oils such as cedar, pine, and cypress have woody aspects that place them in this category. Woody scents are great because they generally blend with almost any other scent category we are discussing in this section. Do keep in mind what my student

Chaplain Nancy Lueschen has found about woody scents: they may not be the best fit for survivors of intimate partner violence.

The heart chakra, anahata, is located in the chest near the heart. It's commonly associated with the thymus gland, which supports healthy immune activity. It's also the seat of unconditional love, healing, and connection to others.

Unresolved trauma can affect the heart chakra, especially when it comes to love for self and others. Trauma can make it difficult to feel connected. Nurturing the heart chakra is an energetic way to help rebuild a sense of healthy relationship with safe people.

Genuine empathy can suffer after witnessing traumatic incidents. This can be a strong reaction, especially if a person feels abandoned or if they are subjected to victim blaming. Unhelpful authority figures, an unsympathetic friend, or judgmental family members can create further traumatic memories that overshadow the helpers.

Nourishing the heart energy can help a person begin to notice the people who were helpful. They will notice those people who are on their side. They will begin to feel supported and protected and can begin supporting others and reconnecting in their own time.

The heart chakra is connected with spicy scents. Cinnamon, nutmeg, and star anise are in this category. Spicy scents blend well with minty, citrus, and floral scents.

The throat chakra, vishuddha, is located in the throat. It is related to the thyroid gland and the voice. A person who has a balanced throat chakra will feel heard and communicate well. Imbalances in the throat chakra can leave a person feeling unheard and undervalued. Some may try to compensate by becoming louder or run over others during the conversation. Others may shrink back and become more invisible.

A person who has been through a traumatic situation may find their throat chakra imbalanced and need support in feeling heard and understood. There are a myriad of ways that someone could deal with a stressful situation and be left with a sense that their voice does not matter. I almost always work the throat chakra together with the third eye, as one's perception is as important as the communication itself.

I associate the throat chakra with minty and camphoraceous scents. Peppermint, spearmint, and eucalyptus all fall into this category. Most of these oils blend well with woody, spicy, fruity, and floral scents.

The third eye chakra, ajna, is superficially located between the brows. Commonly associated with perception and intuition, this chakra is an important energy center for someone recovering from a traumatic situation. It's also connected to the pineal gland, which causes me to work with it anytime someone is struggling with sleep.

A person with unresolved trauma may feel out of touch with their intuition. They may have feelings of not being able to trust themselves, their decisions, or their perception of things that are happening around them. They may even feel they cannot plan for their future. When supporting the third eye chakra through aromatherapy blends as a complementary method, my clients have made amazing progress around these feelings.

Sleep may also be affected when a person is dealing with trauma. Insomnia is a commonly reported issue when the nervous system is affected. I love adding third eye essential oils, along with appropriate herbal support, to support a person who needs higher quality sleep. Because of the uplifting and energizing nature of many of these oils, I tend to recommend them to be used in the morning to help a person's body readjust to a more natural circadian rhythm.

The third eye chakra is associated with citrus scents. Sweet orange, lemon, and grapefruit scents fall into this category. Citrus scents blend well with most woody, spicy, minty, and floral essential oils.

The crown chakra, sahasrara, is located at the top of the head like a crown. It is associated with the pituitary gland: the master gland of the endocrine system. It also is said to govern your connection to the divine. Receiving inspiration toward your higher purpose and feeling connected to something greater than yourself are emotions associated with the crown chakra.

Feeling disconnected from your true calling is common in people who have experienced trauma. Questioning belief systems, feeling cut off from the divine, and struggling to maintain a feeling of purpose is a normal reaction. As a trauma-informed herbalist, your job is not to try to convert clients to a different religion or change their thoughts on the divine. It is to nurture them so they can repair their crown chakra. This can help them come out on the other side of their healing journey with a renewed sense of hope, and possibly even a whole new definition of higher purpose and divine connection.

The crown chakra is associated with floral scents. Palmarosa, lavender, and geranium are all floral scents that help balance the crown chakra. Floral scents blend well with woody, spicy, minty, or fruity scents.

Essential oil safety

This book is not an aromatherapy book, so I do not have enough space to dig as deeply into this topic as I would like. However, I do feel that I need to make a couple of comments on safety. I work with my students in depth on safety training and I encourage you to familiarize yourself with appropriate dilution ratios and application procedures for each oil.

Essential oils are highly concentrated extracts from plants. They are natural and very beneficial in the right circumstances, but should also be respected for their potency and possible contraindications. Below is a brief overview of how I utilize oils in my practice in order to support as many people as possible.

Inhalation is my preferred method of delivery for essential oils. A couple of drops of a blend on a cotton ball can have amazing therapeutic effects. I have small personal inhalers the size of a lipstick tube for clients who enjoy having their oils available on the go. Inhalation is the safest, most reliable way of using aromatherapy.

Diffusion is something that I do not utilize in my practice space, but some people may find it helpful at home. An ultrasonic diffuser allows oils to be dispersed throughout the space and allows anyone in the vicinity to enjoy them. Diffusion should be limited to only a few minutes at a time. This is a great option for private homes with no animals or small children, but I disagree with using them in a practice or in group settings.

Because I have seen people triggered by the smell of different oils, I have stopped diffusing them in my office. Initially I quit using them only in group settings. Then, I began to see one of my clients who struggled every session. When I asked about it, she told me there were smells that were bothering her. We were fragrance free in the session, but the lingering diffusion from the previous sessions was making it difficult for her to feel comfortable in the space.

If you have good ventilation and are able to air out your space in between sessions, then maybe continuing with a diffuser is for you. I still recommend avoiding diffusion in group settings. Whatever you choose, remember it is about what will make your clients most comfortable - not what you think should make them comfortable.

Topical application of essential oils can be a wonderful delivery system. When dilution ratios are appropriate and when care is taken with phototoxic oils, topical application can be generally safe. Make sure you learn safety information about each oil you choose to utilize in your practice.

I do not recommend ever suggesting that a client ingest essential oils. In my integrative aromatherapy research, I have never seen a situation where ingestion of essential oils created a better benefit than utilizing a combination of topical essential oils and internal whole herb extracts. Ingestion has more risks than benefits and ethical herbalists should not be encouraging ingestion in their practice unless they have in-depth clinical aromatherapy training.

Final thoughts

When utilized appropriately, aromatherapy is a strong healing tool for a trauma-informed herbalist. Many people benefit from the different scents available. When an herbalist allows a person to pick their essential oils, the results can be even more powerful.

Aromatherapy is also extremely helpful because it so easily complements many other modalities we may choose to use. In the next chapter, we are discussing flower essences. Flower essences have many complementary emotional healing aspects and pair wonderfully with aromatherapy.

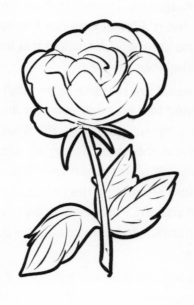

Chapter 11
Flower Essences

The majority of my work as a practitioner is focused on energetic connection. I teach herbalism with a significant focus on the underlying energetics. Therefore, flower essences hold a special place in my heart. Flower essence therapy is the nexus of plant medicine and energetic medicine; it is the purest form of healing art that combines the two.

Flower essences are extracts of (mostly) flowers that have then been diluted into an energetic preparation that is similar to a homeopathic substance. As the flowers are extracted into the water, they are offering vibrational patterns that the water then holds on to. When we dilute a mother tincture, we are further separating the physical aspects from the ethereal, vibrational pattern. Flower essence practitioners believe that this separation helps to create the purest form of vibrational medicine.

Because there is no physical aspect of the flower remaining, flower essences are one of the safest forms of plant-based healing. There are no contraindications and no medication interactions that one must memorize. Most people tolerate flower essences well. The main adjustment I find myself making is to change how often a person is taking their essence.

Creating flower essences

Making your own flower essences is a relatively simple process. The complexity and nuance comes from the ceremonies you can build around the basic processes. I encourage you to experiment with this and find the ways that you connect strongly with the plants you are harvesting.

The number of ceremonies one can use is almost limitless. Some herbalists plan their essence-creating activities around certain celestial events. Others have songs they sing or words they chant. Candles, meditations, poems, music… There are an infinite number of possibilities for plant connection rituals.

Request permission to pick your flowers from the plant and do not take more than is necessary to make the mother tincture. This creates a mindful connection between you and the plant spirit. Whether or not you believe there is a sentient energy to each plant species, this is an important step. Recognizing the need to be conscientious of your consumption is a practice that benefits both you and the plant.

Being able to gather while there is still dew on the plants may add an ethereal quality to the flower essence that may not be available if the flowers are gathered later in the day. Heidi Smith, MA, RH (AHG), points out the added benefits of gathering during the early morning hours in her book The Bloom Book. She highlights Masaru Emoto's work with water consciousness and points out that Dr. Bach considered morning dew to possess important healing properties. If you find yourself drawn to it, try gathering the flowers and beginning your essences first thing in the morning.

Traditionally, flower buds are gathered in the morning as they first begin to open, then are soaked for a few hours under the light of the sun. I have observed that this brings a more action-oriented, "yang" energy to the essence. This can be great when someone needs encouragement to act in order to rebalance.

However, sometimes it can be appropriate to gather flowers at night. Night-blooming flowers may have a better energy when gathered in the evening. In general, night time soaks bring a more contemplative, "yin" energy to the essence. This can be wonderful when someone turns inward to become more aware of their actions and emotions.

Once the flowers have soaked for a few hours, strain the flowers out of the water and pour it into a bottle. Add an equal amount of brandy or glycerin to preserve. Shake, or succuss, for several seconds to thoroughly mix the solution. Some people choose to succuss a certain number of times, usually a symbolic number that reinforces their intention. The resulting liquid is called a mother tincture.

From this mother tincture, you can create a stock bottle. Stock bottles are created by taking a 2 oz bottle and filling it with equal parts water and brandy (or glycerin). Put five drops of the mother tincture into this bottle. Succuss the mixture according to your custom.

Now we dilute the essence one more time. This final dilution is called a dosage bottle. This final dilution usually has a bit more water than alcohol or glycerin. I tend to use 40% alcohol/glycerin, 60% water. Create this mixture, then put five drops of the stock bottle into the dosage bottle. Succuss accordingly, then use in whatever way you find to be most helpful.

How to use flower essences

Flower essences are traditionally used in drop doses under the tongue. Three to four drops are taken three times per day. I adjust this based on a person's needs: sometimes the initial rebalancing effects may be more potent than is comfortable, so we will choose to scale back to only once or twice per day.

Because the vibrational patterns of the flowers are held in water, putting these three to four drops into a glass of water is also a useful option. You may find you have clients that even like to add it to their tea. These three to four drops will create a vibrational pattern throughout the glass, and as you drink you'll get a sensation of a subtle energy shift.

In a similar vein, herbalists have been known to add flower essences to their tinctures. I love to add drops of flower essences into a blend of herbs that are known to support a beneficial emotional state. It cuts down on the cost to the client, and the energetic benefits do not appear to interfere with the energies of the plants in the herbal tincture.

Adding drops of flower essence to a bath can create a sense of peace and gentle balance. Just dropping 5-6 drops into a bath is enough. There are also more intricate ways of using flower essences for the bath. For instance, I like to create bath fizzies with flower essences, physical herbs, and essential oils for support. Explore this: see what you find to be meaningful for you and your clients.

A note on research

Because I studied research so extensively in the Master's of Public Health program I attended, I am fascinated by looking at how complementary modalities are studied. I am also beginning to realize how poorly our natural and traditional modalities are handled in many "high quality" research settings. While they may have a good placebo controlled, double blind structure in place, I do not believe most researchers are aware of how to recommend flower essences for effective application.

For instance, I've seen research where they attempt to apply Rescue Remedy to alleviate test anxiety. Now, I'm not saying there aren't some people who have significant distress at testing events, but I don't believe that Rescue Remedy is an across the board option for addressing anxiety around testing. That kind of overgeneralization of application is bound to get a "no better than placebo" result every time.

So for those of you who are research nerds, I beg you! Start finding ways you can research an essence within its suggested parameters. See if there are different ways to build your research to allow for different underlying constitutions or emotional patterns. Get creative and help us understand more accurately when these flower essences can make a difference for our clients.

The history of Bach Flower Remedies

The idea of energetic preparations that work on the body is not new. The idea of looking to a plant to see what soil it grows in, whether it is in the sun or shade, and what colors or shapes may define its therapeutic values is a concept used by healers around the globe for millenia. While the Bach Remedies we discuss in this chapter are popular options, there are many other plant energy systems that are just as powerful.

When Dr. Bach began looking into how to heal emotional wounds, he was inspired by homeopathy. Homeopathic substances were energetic preparations created by Dr. Samuel Hahnemann to help the body come back into alignment and heal its physical ailments. He believed that by harnessing the subtle energy signature, we could support healing for many without chemicals. His work focused mostly on curing physical ailments.

Dr. Edward Bach had studied homeopathy and began to experiment with how we could use these energy signatures to support people on an emotional level. He believed that healing on an emotional level was integral for a body to return to a fully healthy state. Dr. Bach developed 38 flower essences, designed for many specific emotional imbalances.

Below we are going to discuss some of the original Bach remedies that I frequently implement for someone who is struggling with unresolved trauma. I like the Bach remedies because many people have heard of them and are willing to try them before other essences. This is only one system, so play with what feels right and then try other systems that you are drawn to.

Bach Remedies for trauma

Below I list remedies that I find helpful to have on hand in a trauma-informed setting. This is roughly half the Bach remedies. Although every Bach remedy could be helpful to everyone at some point, I have found these particular options to be beneficial for trauma-informed herbalists. If you find yourself particularly drawn to flower essences, I encourage you to take this inspiration and run with it. They are an amazing source of gentle support.

Rescue Remedy is a blend of several Bach essences that is commonly utilized after a sudden shock or event. When I worked at 911 dispatch, I kept a similar blend on hand for use after difficult calls. The traditional blend consists of Cherry Plum, Clematis, Impatiens, Rock Rose, and Star of Bethlehem.

Rescue remedy is something to consider for any herbal first aid kit. It is also great for doctors, nurses, firefighters, police officers, social workers, or anyone who might be consistently exposed to traumatic situations. I even know a couple of therapists who keep this essence in their office to take after tough sessions.

Agrimony is the essence that shines light on the underlying problems. Commonly given to a person who hides their troubles beneath a façade of happiness. This person may be desperate to never be alone with their feelings.

Numbing repressed emotions can come in many forms. While some turn to alcohol or drugs, less obvious addictions can be just as emotionally damaging. I use Agrimony to help people find the strength to face the repressed emotions as they are brought to light.

Aspen is for a vague sense of foreboding or anxiety that something is going to happen. This general sense of unease perpetually follows you around. You may struggle to know what to do to regain a sense of security.

Clients that tend to need Aspen cannot pinpoint what their fear is about. Many clients who have cases of complex trauma may have these general anxieties without having a direct correlation to one particular root cause. Aspen can bring back the ability for a person to define where the fear is emanating from, or it may bring a sense of security and alleviate the fear altogether.

One final note on Aspen clients: a general sense of unease can also sometimes suggest an underlying physical concern. On occasion, I will have a client who is hesitant to see a conventional medicine physician. If they show signs of foreboding with no apparent cause, I will encourage them to see a doctor to rule out any possible physical issues that are lurking while we are working together on the emotional and vibrational levels.

Beech is for those who have lost sight of the good that still exists in the world. Commonly they tend to be highly critical of everyone and have lost sight of the humanity of the people they criticize. They have become hardened in an attempt to safeguard themselves from further disappointment or pain.

Trauma can cause a person to struggle to see hope or beauty on this plane of existence. Being critical can be a protective mechanism for someone after a horrendous event, especially if it was perpetrated by someone close to them. Beech helps clients to regain a sense of empathy and connectedness that allows them to soften and become more open to trusting others once more.

Cerato is for when we no longer trust our own judgment. We may make choices, but they don't feel like confident decisions. Commonly the clients I see that benefit from Cerato tend to have chameleon-like tendencies to blend in with their friend groups. They may also spend a lot of time trying to get others' opinions on a situation - as if they need validation for the decisions they've made.

I see a need for Cerato most often in people who have been in abusive relationships. Especially for those who chose the relationship and feel they ignored red flags about their abuser. The gaslighting that may occur can lead a person to begin to believe they do not have the ability to execute good decisions. Combine this with external judgments from people who do not understand ("But why did you stay?" "How did you get stuck in this to begin with?"), and it can become an overwhelming sensation of "I don't have good judgment".

Cerato begins to allow people to pay more attention to the decisions they have made that were successful. I have clients return after taking Cerato for a month and they can list off all the ways in which they made good judgment calls over the past few weeks. It opens their eyes to the possibility that they were not responsible for someone else's choice to abuse them.

Cherry Plum is for people who are in the midst of chaos and they are worried that they're going to have an extreme reaction to stress. When we worry we will lose control and do something damaging under pressure, Cherry Plum can help. It can also be helpful if someone has already lost control and responded poorly to a situation.

I regularly use Cherry Plum with many of my clients who find themselves frozen in moments of stress. They are freezing not out of fear of the stressor itself, but from the worry that they might overreact and create a worse situation. Cherry Plum can help a person feel that they have a better sense of an appropriate reaction. It can also help them stay in a cooler state in order to make better decisions in the moment.

Clematis is for when we find ourselves with our head in the clouds. In an everyday situation, Clematis is indicated when someone is prone to daydreaming about how the present or future could be (unrealistically) better. The same grounding energies that bring a person back from this obtrusive daydreaming could be helpful for people with unresolved trauma.

I find myself drawn to suggesting Clematis to clients who report persistent symptoms of dissociation. Their mind has wandered and they cannot ground in the here and now. They're in the same dream-like state of the daydreamer, just as an extreme coping mechanism their brain has enacted to avoid dealing with the feelings of stress their body is producing.

Clematis can bring these people back to a more grounded place. I tend to blend it with other essences that support whatever else a person is struggling with. For instance, Agrimony for clarity or Rock Rose for a feeling of jittery-ness.

Gorse is indicated for the times when we have given up all sense of hope to the point where we reject anyone's attempts at consolation. We may actively argue against any suggestion that things could become better. We have succumbed to a feeling of helplessness and no longer have an interest in finding a way out.

I reach for Gorse when someone is living through a chronically traumatic situation or has experienced some form of complex trauma and is ready to give up. It is also one that I may use when someone who has a chronic illness begins to lose hope from the uncertainty and traumatic experiences related to their disease. I find it particularly effective when the person is no longer showing strong emotions such as despair; they are just existing and have no capacity to see a different way forward.

Gorse can help our clients consider other aspects that can restore hope. It helps people begin to entertain other ideas and pull out of the extreme stagnation that lack of motivation creates. It may not fix the situation, but it empowers a person to begin finding their way back.

Impatiens is a teacher of acceptance. It is commonly utilized when someone's impatience causes them to become agitated. Impatiens encourages someone to slow down and stop forcefully willing the future into the now.

A state of hyperarousal can lead a person to become restless and irritable. Agitation can be calmed when Impatiens is utilized. I reach for this when clients are struggling to become mindfully aware of this moment and instead find themselves obsessing about what comes next.

Larch is helpful to encourage us to continue making progress, even when we feel likely to fail. It creates a sense of inner resilience and motivation. It allows us to persevere without being as concerned with outside influences.

This is my "vulnerability essence". When someone has been through a trauma, has begun to recover, and they are still struggling with being vulnerable in relatively safe environments, I reach for Larch. Note: If someone is still in the early stages of trauma recovery, I spend time helping them foster a sense of safety before suggesting Larch.

Mustard is indicated when we are drowning in sadness or despair that seems to unexpectedly descend. We may be able to see why we *should* feel better, but in the moment the sadness is too overwhelming. Mustard can help bring back a sense of contentment and peace.

Like Larch, Mustard is another "recovery phase" flower essence. Initially I want to look at behaviors and plan specific essences to support the person's response to unresolved trauma. However, once they begin to recover, an unexpected bout of despair can be a sign of lingering energetic or emotional imbalance that can be released through using Mustard essence.

Pine relieves the unnecessary guilt that comes with a strong inner critic. It is useful especially when we're doing mental gymnastics to blame ourselves for something that could not possibly be our fault. Pine helps to create discernment between the things we should correct and the things we do not control.

Many times complex trauma patients have this strong inner critic that beats them up, but that may not be something they divulge. Therefore we should look for other signs, such as strong negative self talk, that indicate more care is needed. Pine is my first choice when a client comes in apologizing for everything - especially if the constant "sorry"s are related to actions that don't warrant an apology.

Rock Rose is for those times when we are jumpy and ill at ease. My mom described the feeling best, when at the beginning of the pandemic she said "it is like we are walking around in a horror movie... perpetually at the point where you have goosebumps in anticipation of the jump scare that is about to occur." That sense of chronic terror is seen in people who have experienced some form of trauma. It became very commonplace here at the beginning of 2020, as America was plunged into lockdown.

When this panicky sensation is a constant companion, someone may struggle to make decisions that are rational and appropriate. Rock Rose brings a sense of calmness and clarity that allows for a respite from the constant skittishness. I use this with almost everyone at some point in their work with me.

Star of Bethlehem is used after a life-altering event. While we normally think of applying this formula when we first have something occur, it can transcend time and support the after effects of shocks that happened years ago. Usually this helps most after a sudden, unexpected event.

Anyone who comes to me with an experience of an acute trauma is going to benefit from Star of Bethlehem. I find it really helpful if I see signs that they haven't been able to integrate the event. These signs could include scattered thoughts, struggling with memories around the event, or being unable to stop talking about the event.

Sweet Chestnut is for a person who is experiencing extreme anguish. You may choose this when you feel you are drowning and have reached the limit of your ability to cope with life's stressors. It's for that moment where you feel you have done everything in your power and yet things continue to crumble around you.

When someone feels they are at the end of their rope, they are unable to see how to keep pushing forward, and are in despair from that thought, I offer them Sweet Chestnut. When a client feels they have been razed to the ground, this essence can bring a renewed sense of strength. This strength can bring about a sense of calm and give a person a chance to feel they can hang on until a new option opens up.

Walnut is for when we are facing changes or are going through the typical transitions of life. New relationships, jobs, and homes can be positive stressors, but even the positive can add extra stress. Walnut helps to buffer any extraneous stress we may face. The resilience offered by this essence is beneficial to us at any point in our life, but has become especially important for my trauma-informed practice.

When someone is healing from trauma, changes are inevitable. When I am able to offer a client Walnut as an ally during this time, the changes feel less daunting. A person's energy is limited after dealing with a traumatic event. Being able to spend that energy on healing and feeling safe instead of adjusting to changes is a big help.

Water Violet is our helper when we need to remember how to foster connection. I am always reminded of the lyrics to the Simon and Garfunkel song, I am a Rock. In the song, the subject boasts of his ability to be an island without friendship and that it keeps him from feeling pain. Sometimes we can feel that it is easier to be isolated than to deal with the strong emotions that come with vulnerability.

Water Violet helps my clients begin to shed this misconception. It allows a person to feel they have the strength to stand in connection with others. Isolation may feel safe in the short term, but connection is the state in which people thrive. Water Violet helps reveal this truth.

Wild Oat is our helper to connect with our purpose and higher calling. When you find yourself wandering, unsure of what you are meant to do, Wild Oat can be your guide. I like to use it before meditation by placing a few drops in my tea.

This may not seem to have a place in trauma-informed care. After all, Maslow's hierarchy of needs suggests that self actualization cannot occur if we are still fighting to maintain a sense of safety and survival. However humans are rarely so linear. I find that sometimes adding Wild Oat to a blend can help a person gain clarity that makes it easier for them to find their right path to healing.

Willow is for those times where we become resentful and bitter. Why are the people around me finding success and I'm still stuck here? Many times we have our own accomplishments, but they are overshadowed by previous injustices.

Please note, I am not suggesting we should brush off injustice. It is always appropriate to protest an unjust situation. I am also not suggesting that a person must forget about systemic discrimination. When we are speaking of Willow's healing properties, they are only freeing us from resentment so we can be better prepared to fight back when necessary.

I find Willow is useful in many traumatic situations. A person may find themselves clouded by the resentment that can occur after a horrible trauma. When someone is stuck in a place of self pity, or struggling to let go of somatic sensations because of resentment they hold, I use this essence. Willow flower essence can help to relieve the unhealthy attitudes toward the traumatic situation and reorient a person to a more productive path.

Exploration and expansion

As with our discussion in the last chapter of essential oils, it is impossible to do flower essences justice with the space I have available in this chapter. While Bach's flower essences were the original essence therapy, there are other effective systems that utilize energetic flower preparations. For instance, the Flower Essence Society has created an amazing repertoire of North American essences that extends our understanding of flower essences well beyond Dr. Bach's English list.

If you find this is something you want to study further, I encourage you to look into other flower essence lists. Learn why each flower essence has been given its corresponding traits. Try some of the essences and see how they feel when you use them. When trying to develop a friendship with a flower, I will work with its essence for about a month.

When it feels right, I invite you to explore flowers that are not codified into a system. Find local plants that grow in your area and connect with them. Make a mother essence from them. Dilute it appropriately and use the flower essence for a month to feel the relationship forming. How could this essence be helpful to you? To your clients? Keep notes and explore the sensations.

Personal flower essences

I want to share with you a few of my own flower essences. These are flowers that I have felt drawn to as I work in my garden. I have mostly created these descriptions from my personal experience.

I offer these less in an attempt to codify the descriptions and more as a way for you to see how I think about the essences. Local flower essences are a powerful option for your clients. I hope that you'll be able to take these ideas and apply similar concepts to your own private flower essence collection.

Passionflower is an interesting plant here, because we have a *Passiflora lutea* that is native to our area. I prefer *lutea* to *incarnata* in my work here. Their essence is similar, but I find the yellow *lutea* flowers have a more calming and energizing feel. The purple *incarnata* flowers are more sedating.

I suggest the *lutea* essence to my busy clients who need to have a chance to relax but also need to keep going. My unique people who are beautiful masterpieces but may need support that they don't currently have. Like the passion flower vine, they need to reach out and find support in the community around them so that they can bloom in their unique ways.

Passionflower accepts that not everyone can leave the kids with grandma, take a spa weekend, and come back refreshed. It offers to take the edge off and make the stress more bearable. Blunting the sharp jab of responsibilities so that everything doesn't feel like a life-or-death situation.

Many of my clients need this when they're trying to juggle home duties, work, and a sense of their own wellness. They may not feel they have time to stop and smell the roses because there is so much they are responsible for. However, it gives them a chance to shift their focus. Bringing them from a place where their nose is to the grindstone to a place where they can look up and around to build community.

Mimosa has the spirit of a happy-go-lucky friend who only wants the best for you. Here in Alabama it blooms in early summer, right as things are getting so hot that you just want to sit around in a daze. The blooms are a bright pink color, usually with a touch of white, and they fan out in an almost "jazz hands" shape. Mimosa helps to pull you out of mild dazes and bring you back to happier things.

I like to use Mimosa when clients are reporting they find themselves zoned out. Not from depression or trying to avoid things, just in a bit of an energy slump. Mimosa has the ability to reach out and lift you from a place of "dazed and confused" into a space of grateful awareness.

Elderflower is another favorite of mine that has a cooling, protective effect. My elderflower plants are happiest in pairs. When you find yourself needing a quiet, strong friend, elderflower will be there.

Elderflower is a five petal flower, so it falls into a category of plants that offer a transition. I find myself using this alongside Walnut for many of my clients who are struggling to get out of traumatic situations. Elderflower helps to remind us that community is a support that carries us through all of life's situations.

Oregon Grape is a new essence that I've only recently started working with, as our new home has an Oregon grape plant at the top of our hill. I have found it has a strong association with my solar plexus. It appears to also hold the key to reintegrating parts of myself that I have rejected for so long out of fear.

As we will discuss in the next chapter, flower essences can be an amazing way to connect with plants. Oregon grape has recently reminded me of how serendipitous our plant encounters can be. We can learn a lot from the plants we are surrounded by, and if we listen hard enough we can even be offered the wisdom for our own healing.

Chapter 12
Plant Spirit
Connection

Plants have a vital life force that heals. This goes beyond the chemical constituents that can be isolated and shown to have physical effects. The ability of plants to offer holistic healing without lots of complexity is such a gift, yet many herbalists don't tap into the power available to us from the plant spirits.

You may have had intuitive moments where you felt the urge to use a plant in an unorthodox fashion. Perhaps you gave in to that intuition and were rewarded with phenomenal results. Moments like these, when you reach for a plant without a full understanding of why - that is a plant spirit connection at work.

All herbalists have some form of a personal relationship with plants. Whether it is just an understanding of the commonly accepted healing traits of a plant or a connection to the plant that is in their garden, that relationship is there. Many healing traditions indicate that we can strengthen these relationships to create phenomenal healing situations.

Do plants have a sentient spirit? I believe so and I contend that there is a conscious spirit attached. But before you roll your eyes and flip to the next chapter, please note that the majority of this information can be applied whether you believe that or not.

Some herbalists choose to see plant spirit connection as their subconscious parsing out useful information about the natural vibrations given off by a plant. Their focus on, or communion with, the plant allows their subconscious to pick up on these energetic signatures. They believe the messages they receive are the result of a subconscious intuitive moment.

However you view it, the information presented here can be applied to help you on your journey to be a more trauma-informed herbalist. You can personally connect with plants for a better understanding of their therapeutic properties. You can encourage others to connect closely with the herbs they are using for deeper meaning. You can even suggest forms of plant spirit connection to clients who are struggling with unresolved trauma, giving them the chance to experience a safe connection with healing energies.

Connecting with the land

Before attempting to connect directly with a plant, I ask you: what is your connection to the land on which you are currently residing? A holistic approach to plant connection should include a conscientious connection to the land. How can you expect unhindered communication to occur if your attitudes toward the land are possessive?

Many people grow up with a sense that the land is there to serve them. They want to get what they can out of the land, without thinking about creating a reciprocal relationship. Rarely do people pay attention to the resonance coming from the land, yet we as herbalists are called to do just that.

I am lucky. I grew up with a grandfather who kept a large garden and great uncles with farms and a respect for their Native American heritage. I watched them treat the land with honor. I was taught to see our home as a responsibility. We were expected to be stewards of the land, doing the best we could to keep the vegetation healthy.

But I cannot rest on the laurels of my forebears. New information is coming out all of the time on how we can do better. I've learned so much over the past few years about no-till methods that keep the microbes in the soil healthier. I know more about companion planting now than I ever learned growing up. So even though I grew up with a general understanding of the land, I am still finding ways to more fully understand my responsibilities.

What can you do to connect to the area you're in? If you are in a city, it might be simply going to a local park. Perhaps volunteering at a community garden. Maybe hiking in the state parks on the weekend.

If you're on a plot of land, what native plants can you reintroduce? How can you make a better environment for the natural wildlife you see? There are so many ways we can start honoring the places in which we live. Find something small and start today.

Ancestor traditions toward the land

When we are looking to connect with the land, there are many traditions that can guide the way. Take time to honor your ancestry and learn the practices that your forebears have used in the past to respect the land. Find a trusted elder that can guide you. Read and focus on others that have a similar path and ancestry.

White people: be cautious when considering your ancestry. Magnifying and glorifying a tiny part of your past can be a temptation. Our privilege puts us in a position where we can easily take things out of context for our benefit. Be cognizant of this and consider carefully when looking at small aspects of your heritage that are overshadowed by the larger tide of colonization and oppression.

While my grandfather and his brothers knew my Indigenous ancestors, I was born forty years after the last of these ancestors passed. I am appreciative of the practices of the Cherokee, but I don't look to showcase their practices in my work. Because my indigenous ancestors have moved on, I don't have the appropriate context to fully embrace their legacy as my own.

Because of this, I mainly look to the Appalachian-esque practices I was taught and I study the Celtic traditions of how the land was respected. When you are looking at your own path, find ways you can respect the land you currently inhibit. Don't let yourself feel constrained to ceremonial work - practical applications such as working to be less wasteful can be a strong way to show your respect for the land.

Friendships with plants

Once you have a comfortable connection to the land, you can begin looking more specifically to individual plants. Emotional healing that comes from plants can be amplified when these relationships are maintained in a healthy manner. This connection encourages more of those subtle, intuitive moments in which you reach for a plant and use it in an unorthodox capacity.

Just like human relationships, some plant energies will resonate more closely with you than others. There may be plants you want to befriend that don't seem interested. Other plants may be begging for your attention and you feel uncertain about that connection. Look for plants that you feel connected to that are receptive to your energy right now.

Once you have some experience with connecting to plant spirits, revisit plants that are calling to you but you were initially hesitant to work with. Sometimes they have lessons for us that we wouldn't otherwise accept. The hesitancy we feel toward them may be an emotional block that they can help us remove.

I've had a recent experience like this with Oregon grape (*Mahonia aquifolium*). When we moved into this house, there was this plant on the hill that was smack dab in the middle of what would be a magnificent clearing. I knew immediately when we viewed the property the first time: I was going to get up there and remove the scraggly bush.

But once I actually walked up the hill and realized what it was, I felt guilty about the idea of tearing it down. Oregon grape has a lot of fantastic medicinal properties and I couldn't let it go to waste. However, I didn't find myself drawn to it, either. It would call to me, offering friendship, but it took me a while to get to a point where I wanted that.

Now I'm grateful for the fact I chose to accept that offer of friendship. Oregon grape has helped me to integrate parts of myself that I was rejecting for fear of others rejecting me. I recently completed a round of its flower essence and it has been an eye opener. I implore you: go ahead and connect with those plants that maybe don't seem as glorious at first glance. Those connections can offer some amazing benefits.

Ways to connect

There are more ways to connect to plants than I have time to address in this chapter. However, I did want to speak to a few of the common ways you may find useful. As with much of this material, this is the tip of the iceberg. I encourage you to take inspiration from this and go down all the rabbit holes.

Speaking or singing to plants is one way to form a connection. Take time every day to spend a few moments with a plant. If you have one growing in your yard that you want to get to know better, sit down with it for a few minutes and tell it about your day. Sing it your favorite song. See if there is a vibe that comes from the plant.

Journal your experience as you continue to form this connection. Are there certain songs that it seems to enjoy? Do you find telling it about certain parts of your day helps you feel more connected? Focusing on noticing where the connection is stronger may lead you to more information about how you will interact with the plant spirit.

Once you've become accustomed to talking to the plant, the inverse is also helpful. Take time and just listen to the intuitive nudges you receive while sitting with the plant. Clear your mind, allowing your focus to be on the plant and its resonance. Many times we spend more time trying to be heard than actively listening - plants provide a safe space to listen and feel secure.

This listening exercise has also caused me to notice more about myself. I notice the days where I am feeling grounded. I can compare them to the feeling of days where I feel jumpy. When I take the time to sit and listen, I notice more about my interaction with my environment and I walk away with a more focused intention for the rest of my day.

Plant meditation can be a part of a focused listening activity. If you have a plant you want to connect with further, spending time reflecting on the plant can bring a familiarity to its resonance that you cannot get otherwise. Softening your gaze, focusing on the plant (a physical plant is best, though a picture will work if a plant is unavailable), and using the plant as an anchor if your mind begins to wander.

Similar to a mindfulness based contemplative practice, this type of plant focused clearing of the mind may help you notice more intuitive nudges. Plants offer safe relationships that allow you to feel connected without concern. They can help you feel more comfortable with subconscious exploration through things like dreamwork.

Dream work can help you to tap into a more subconscious space to find deeper meaning and connection with plant energies. I like to drink a cup of tea that contains the plant I'm working with right before bedtime. With more potent plants (especially the poisonous ones) I'll use flower essences. Tinctures can also work with edible plants. You are just looking for a way to strengthen the connection as you begin to enter your dream world.

When you wake up in the morning, take a few moments to record your dreams. Before you ever leave the bed, grab your notebook and pen and jot down what you remember. Too many times I have jumped up to handle something, promising myself that I would remember the dream details for later, only to realize that afternoon that I couldn't remember any of it.

While dreamwork may not immediately bear fruit, there are elements of self observation that will begin to emerge. As you continue to work with different plants, there may be different dream segments that you can attribute to a certain plant. This leaves room for a lot of interpretation, but my belief is those dream segments can help you to discover more about your relationship with said plant.

Dreamwork is an interesting prospect for connecting to plants through the subconscious, but guided meditation can lead us in a similar direction with a bit more structure. Record your own guided meditations or find one that speaks to you. I take my students on guided meditations to find plant spirit connections frequently, and it is usually a productive journey.

Some of these aspects might be helpful for clients. Guided meditation is a common way to tap into some of these intuitive connections to plants. Please refer to the next chapter on mindfulness and meditation for my tips on how to lead a successful guided meditation in a trauma-informed environment.

Plants in your ancestor traditions

Back to the subject of honoring your ancestry: are there certain plants that are part of your ancestry?

Indigenous tribes used many of the plants native to their area. Each tribe had different ways of working with their local plants. It can benefit you to learn more about your ancestral tribes and the plants they worked with on a regular basis.

American slavery brought over many traditions that were then disseminated in many forms of healing practices. If you have ancestry that includes people who were stolen from their native African lands, explore the ways their plants were used. Look into the work done by Emma Dupree and learn more about the Black Herbalism Movement.

Asian cultures have amazing ancestral traditions. Even Scottish herbal traditions remain in several Highland folk traditions. Take time to look into your ancestry and connect to some of the plants your ancestors might have used.

Recommendations and ego

Your plant spirits may lead you to use certain plants or remedies that don't quite make sense. Sometimes these nudges can come into play when we are working with clients. I encourage you to follow those nudges if the intuitive recommendations you are feeling are safe and not contraindicated for the person.

Note these recommendations and notice the results you are getting. If they are generally positive, there is a good chance you're connecting well to the plant energy. If they are neutral or negative, there may be some ego issues hindering your connection.

Releasing ego is one of the hardest things to do as a practitioner. There are pieces of our psyche that want to be recognized for the hard work we are doing. We want to be right, and sometimes our insecurities can cause us to worry about whether or not someone will recognize our expertise.

We may compare ourselves to herbalists that we think are well known or more popular. It can be demoralizing to get into that space of measuring ourselves against people who have made more important contributions (or at least that's how we see it). In turn, your thoughts may be muddled and your intuition may be diverted by emotion.

When we are struggling with ego, many things can be out of balance. Ego can cause us to desperately want to be seen as right and we may push a point or misrepresent a recommendation. On the other end of the ego reaction spectrum, we may second guess our intuition and miss out on an opportunity to help someone. This is why I say, if your intuitive recommendations seem to be more often wrong than right, look to your ego and see where the problem lies.

When we start working with others in such a capacity, we must keep this in mind. Many people have seriously hurt others by recommendations that common sense indicates are not safe. Many times these people truly believe they are right in recommending these things - which indicates to me that there may be an ego issue at play.

When we find ego creeping in during a consult, the easiest thing to do is recognize it and respond accordingly. Shift your focus to your clients. Focus on only tangible recommendations. Leave intuition for another day when your head is more clear.

Plant communion for trauma support

You can always find ways to encourage your clients to connect with nature. I have found that these connections provide a safe, relatively relaxing space for most people. We can offer many low cost options for plant communion that help everyone, and can be twice as helpful if someone is struggling with unresolved trauma.

Can this relationship we are cultivating with plants really lead to a calmer, more secure state? I believe so. The consistent nature of our relationship with plants can lead us into healing before we are able to find that same support in the human realm.

When a client comes to me with trauma, I may recommend some sort of plant communication. I will usually spare them the philosophizing that I've done with you in this chapter, but I will recommend some form of connection to nature. Almost every time I do this, my clients find some way to connect more deeply with their surroundings.

Forest bathing is usually a well received recommendation. Many people benefit from taking a leisurely walk in the woods with the only focus being to become more attuned to nature. Especially if someone's natural tendency is to walk with purpose to their destination, taking time to slow down and mindfully connect with each step can bring healing opportunities that they might otherwise miss.

Gardening is another fantastic, hands-on option for people who are struggling with trauma. Besides the zen nature of tending to plants, the benefits of being outside and in the dirt make this a wonderful option to recommend. I love suggesting plants that are easy to grow and can be used in teas or food.

Rosemary, peppermint, lemon balm, or thyme could be good starter plants.

Many people see gardening as an expensive endeavor - our capitalistic society has made it seem like you need hundreds of dollars of soil modifiers and equipment to be a successful gardener. While these things can be useful, they aren't required for a lovely garden. Low cost gardening options may not be readily apparent to your clients. If you feel led to encourage gardening, designing a handout with information about low cost gardening could help your clients get started.

Guided meditations can be a good option for leading someone to become more connected to plants. However there are some considerations that need to be taken into account if you're recommending meditation when someone has unresolved trauma. The next chapter will dig into more of when mindfulness practices and meditation can be useful - and when these options have the capacity to further traumatize.

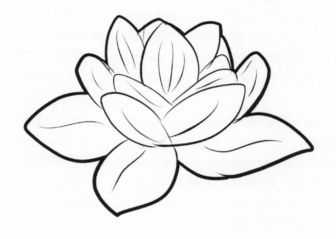

Chapter 13
Mindfulness and
Meditation

Many herbalists practice some form of meditation, guided journeys, or mindfulness techniques with their clients. Mindfulness is the practice of being conscious and aware of your body and mind in the present moment. While Mindfulness Based Stress Reduction (MBSR) techniques and mindfulness meditation tend to be the most commonly recognized forms of mindfulness, there are other, less formalized tools that can be helpful.

Meditation encompasses a wider range of practices that help to train the mind in focus and awareness. This can include practices such as vipassana, yoga nidra, or mindfulness meditation. Different forms of meditation may help people with unresolved trauma, but sometimes people struggle with being still and silent for long periods of time.

In this chapter, we explore different mindfulness practices, different meditation techniques, and what to do when someone is uncomfortable with these practices. There are many ways to adapt mindfulness and meditation practices to fit someone's needs. Remember, no one system is required for a person to experience healing. Our job as trauma informed herbalists is to find the right combination of support for each client.

The healing power of meditation

Meditation gives us a chance to slow down and enter a calm, relaxed state. It also can help us access subconscious healing thoughts and experiences. We can use compassion practices and other guided, contemplative practices to help us further train our brain for healthy responses. The healing effects that can occur make meditation a frequently encouraged practice.

Mindfulness meditation brings us into a space where we can become aware of our bodies and the signals we are being given. Generally this is helpful to bring a person into better tune with their needs. Mindfulness, when practiced for a long period of time, can help a person notice when they have left that ventral vagal state of safety. Then they can use the techniques they've learned to more quickly bring them back into that connected place.

Encouraging clients to notice physical sensations can help them become more in tune with what their body is telling them. Paying attention to those moments and being able to describe what is happening can give them more tools to work with whatever is coming up. They can take these observations back to their therapist and find ways to process through the narrative that these sensations may create.

Once my clients and students are able to notice and describe these sensations, we move on to determining whether we are reacting or responding. In my trauma-informed groups, I don't use this as a gauge for whether or not someone is doing it "right". Instead, I encourage people to notice whether they can switch reactions to responses. If they can, then we continue to notice when we are able to change a reaction into a response. When they can't, I have them note those moments and take them to their therapist to discuss why that may be happening.

I hope to lead clients to a place where they can experience things in equanimity. I want them to eventually be able to move into the role of conscious observer, even when they are feeling distressed. Play with these different ideas for yourself: when can you change your reaction into a response? When it is something you may need therapeutic support to address?

Language of guided meditation

Guided meditations are a wonderful option for many people to experience a chance to journey into their subconscious. Our language when facilitating these meditations can make a difference for someone's experience. Of course, the language considerations we discussed in chapter five will always apply. However, there are certain things that could be helpful to consider when looking at a guided experience.

Reconsider making blanket statements. Broad ideas such as "you are always safe" could cause a person to feel uncertain or activated. I prefer to say "notice what parts of your body feel safe and relaxed at this moment." It is more concrete and less likely to lead someone to feeling uneasy.

If you are directing someone's attention to different parts of their body, be conscious of how a person might feel toward those parts. Some people may have experiences that make them uncomfortable if we focus on the mouth, tongue, or throat. When someone is struggling with food, "stomach" or "tummy" could be activating - try using "abdomen" instead.

Consider how you will approach each section of your meditation. For most of us, the beach is a relaxing setting. However, for someone who experienced a trauma on a beach, it may not be where they feel safest. How do you prepare for this? We cannot poll each student before class to get their deepest, darkest fears. Even if we could, some people might not realize they are going to react to a beach scene.

In a trauma-informed setting, I always tell students what we will be focused on during meditation. I walk them through each of the settings and a general overview of the purpose of that setting. That way, there are no surprises when moving from one scene to the next. This cuts down on the number of unexpected shifts that could cause a person to feel unsafe.

Check in after class. Keep time open so that you can observe everyone as they are leaving. Give people the chance to speak with you in case someone has questions or feedback. If anyone mentions being activated by a certain phrase or scene, take that information into consideration as you build future meditations.

Mindful acceptance is not approval

When practicing mindfulness, we sometimes reference an idea of accepting sensations, pain, or emotions as they come. Mindfulness Based Stress Reduction techniques even go so far as to say we "befriend" the sensations that feel negative. We work to notice these sensations without struggling against the experience. In a trauma-informed setting, the idea of acceptance is meant to be a neutral feeling toward the sensations and emotions that arise.

This idea of "acceptance" can be misconstrued by newcomers to your class as a directive to embrace negative events or sensations. This can make a person uncomfortable, and understandably so. How can you be expected to enjoy chronic pain? Why would we try to encourage a positive response to trauma flashbacks?

To try to reduce the misinterpretations of "acceptance", I frequently discuss the ideas of passive observation and neutrality in my mindfulness groups. I work to define mindful acceptance as a place of equanimity, not toxic positivity. If you incorporate these ideas into your meditation circles and become aware of other language that might cause someone distress, you will be more successful at supporting people with unresolved trauma.

Meditation is not a cure-all

Mindfulness meditation has been marketed as an infallible relaxation technique that will create a perfect, stress free environment for anyone who practices long enough. However the reality is not so simple. Unresolved trauma can cause a person to struggle significantly with mindfulness meditation practices.

I loved meditation and mindfulness practices, but once I experienced my own trauma I struggled with mindfulness work. When I started volunteering at UAB hospital's integrative clinic, I was baffled at my body's reaction to the mindfulness meditation classes. I would anxiously come to the clinic, be able to help in early classes, but then mindfulness would knock the breath out of me.

I couldn't focus on being present. I would start listening for sounds around us that indicated we were in danger. The room only had one door in and out, so I would start trying to think how we could create a barricade if we needed to protect ourselves.

Coming back to focus on my breath would make me worry about having a panic attack. I was mortified by the idea of becoming the center of attention and taking away from the patients who were there to cope with greater struggles than I could imagine. More than once I would have to leave the room.

I am forever grateful to the way the facilitator, Dr. Mark, approached my situation. She walked with me several times after class, talking to me and helping me regulate. I never felt shamed for leaving the group when necessary and her willingness to skillfully guide me through the sensations of trauma that were triggered was an integral part of my ability to continue pursuing mindfulness meditation practices.

My hope is that you can recognize when a client is struggling and help them figure out a better path. While Dr. Mark had a multitude of therapy tools that aren't available to herbalists, it was her ability to help me understand that my PTSD was being exacerbated by the practice that made the biggest difference. She helped me to recognize what I needed in order to move forward and get the healing that set me back on track.

Mindfulness meditation is generally an enjoyable practice, but there are times in which the inward focus is not well tolerated. People who are struggling with unresolved trauma are on high alert. Their body is watching for signs of danger and they may be more likely to gravitate toward negative sensations and memories.

The most common concern I have is that when one of my clients slows down, they may start noticing sensations and remembering experiences they were not ready to face. Many mindfulness practices are designed to help us understand more about who we are without outside influences, but if someone is still in the early stages of healing from trauma they may find this to be disorienting.

Mindfulness meditation in trauma-informed care

As with most natural healing practices, meditation is not an all-or-nothing situation. Different clients will need different support systems in order to receive the healing that is offered. As trauma-informed herbalists, we remain committed to finding new ways to adjust sessions for the benefit of all our clients.

There are many different accommodations that can be made in meditation practices to help people feel as safe as possible. Your job as facilitator is to learn different ways you can shift the practice and then make sure to communicate these adjustments to your clients. Verbal permission and reminders can help them begin to incorporate these accommodations to meet their needs.

Traditional meditation postures and techniques may not work for everyone - and that's OK. We can benefit from sitting quietly and keeping our eyes open. Some people may prefer to lie down throughout meditation, others may need permission to sit up if they become activated. Healing can still occur if someone focuses on the music playing instead of their breathing. Some people may even benefit from shorter sessions at first.

When I bring someone into a meditative state, I encourage them to soften their gaze and then close their eyes if it feels right. This gives people permission to leave their eyes open if that is more comfortable. At the end of the session, I always bring people back by saying something like "if your eyes are closed, you may open them, and bring your gaze back into focus." This keeps it from feeling as if the default must be eyes shut.

Meditation can be practiced in a variety of positions. I always let people know that they can stay in a seated position, find a comfortable restorative yoga pose, or lie down. I also make sure people know that they are allowed to quietly change positions at any time during the meditation.

There is a balance to be had for the amount of movement you allow in a stationary meditation session. I do request that participants stay on their mat throughout the meditation. If a person is relaxed and has their eyes closed, this can feel open and vulnerable. Another participant getting up and moving around could be startling or activating.

Some people struggle with stationary meditation. I do not encourage people to push through uncomfortable feelings during meditation. Instead, I help them find ways to adapt and change their meditation practice for their needs. Shorter meditations to introduce them to the stillness can be helpful.

If someone tells you that they struggle within the first five minutes of a class, encourage them to start with thirty seconds. The idea is to meditate below that threshold, grasping those moments of ventral vagal activation, and walking away with a positive feeling. Then when they come back, they may try for 45 seconds. Then for a minute… knowing that they can reduce the time if they begin feeling activated at any point.

Walking meditations can also be used. Slowly walking in a circle is a common form of walking meditation. During a walking meditation, a person may choose to focus on their breathing or they may focus on the sensation of the floor connecting with their feet. This connection can have a grounding feel that may be welcome if someone is struggling to feel present during meditative practice.

Labyrinths are another walking meditation tool that can be useful. I love walking the labyrinth near our house, feeling a sense of focus on the moment as I weave around the center. I love a Chartres-style labyrinth, as the extra twists and turns help keep me from being able to anticipate what is next. Instead, I am able to focus in the moment on my steps, allowing myself to be swept along to the center without a plan.

Mindful tea

One of my favorite forms of practicing mindfulness is to have mindful tea time. This is a practice that utilizes focusing on the act of drinking tea in order to stay focused in the moment. Assuming the tea is a flavor and smell that your client enjoys, this practice is a relatively well-tolerated option to orient people into the present.

Beginning with a cup of tea that is steeping, notice the smell of the tea. Notice the warmth of the cup on your hands. Notice the color changing as it brews.

Once the tea is ready to drink, continue to notice the smell. Take small sips and notice the taste. The entire experience can become a mindfulness practice. Are there astringent herbs that are leaving a toning sensation in your mouth? As it cools, does the taste change? How do you begin to feel as your body begins absorbing the herbs?

If you practice this every day around the same time, you can start to notice subtle changes in your body. This does not have to be a time consuming habit. Stopping for twenty minutes and checking in with yourself can help you to pivot your activities based on what is going to be most supportive to you.

Breath focus and other anchors

In most mindfulness classes, the aim is to focus on the movement of the breath, in and out of the body. For many people, this is a soothing activity. But for many others, focusing on the breath can activate a sense of being unsafe. There are a variety of medical, socio-political, and domestic violence situations that can cause a person to later struggle with focusing on their breath.

When someone struggles with breath as a safe anchor, all is not lost. There are other senses that can be employed in order to refocus into the present moment. Music, touching the thumb to another finger, the smell of a favorite essential oil, or focusing on a single spot can be safe anchors for students.

Focusing on the music allows a person to return to the present through the sense of sound. Some people find this method is a helpful anchor during meditation. I encourage you to find instrumental music that doesn't include popular tunes to make it a safe option for clients.

Finger tracing helps a person to come back to the present through the sense of touch. You can encourage people to touch their thumb to their fingers and notice that sensation when they need to come back to the present moment. I have also found that alternating sides (touching my left thumb to my left fingers, then touching my right thumb to my right fingers, and repeat) creates a comforting, bilateral aspect to the practice.

If a person has a particular essential oil they enjoy, having a personal inhaler on them during practice can give them a way to anchor through the sense of scent. I frequently have blends or single oils on hand for my clients to use if they prefer this method of anchoring. I have even had some students use it as a way to reintroduce breathwork into their practice as they begin to heal. The essential oil feels calming and reassuring as they inhale and they can focus on that feeling of safety anytime the breath feels activating.

Focusing on a specific spot while meditating can be helpful as an anchor. This allows a person to come to the present through visual cues. I don't use this one as often in practice, but some people find it the easiest option for connection. Clients can pick a spot on the wall, or you can offer intentional visual anchors. One way I do use visual anchors is through candle gazing

Candle gazing is used in a variety of metaphysical practices. For mindfulness meditations, my interest is encouraging people to stay present in the flickering of the flame. Focusing in the present on something that dances without a pattern helps us to stay in the moment without anticipating the next.

More informal meditative practices can be helpful, especially if someone struggles to sit through a traditional silent meditation. I've offered meditation classes built around adult coloring sessions. Having people focus on the very spot where their pencil is at any given time may seem ineffective at first glance, but being brought into that present moment can help bring people into a ventral vagal state of calm.

This is not an exhaustive list. Introduce different ideas for safe anchors to clients and let them see what works best for them. Brainstorm ideas with other trauma-informed practitioners in your area. The more creative you get, the more ways you will have to adjust a session if someone is struggling!

A note on spiritual healing traditions

Similarly to mindfulness meditations, other forms of turning inward can be extremely difficult for a client in the early stages of trauma healing. If I can see a person's window of tolerance is extremely low, I avoid some of the techniques that I love - including Yoga Nidra, Reiki-only sessions, and restorative yoga - until they feel more secure in their practice. Introducing these practices earlier than necessary and risking a retraumatization event is not worth it - no matter what healing benefits they theoretically could receive.

Sometimes I hear people talk about the traumatic sensations they have experienced during meditation practices as if they are spiritual awakenings. Some practitioners indicate that pushing through these uncomfortable sensations will lead us to some form of higher consciousness breakthrough. This is a dangerous view to take, as pushing someone to continue experiencing flashbacks and trauma related symptoms during meditation can cause a person to experience hypo arousal or a dissociation state.

Many herbal traditions combine some form of spiritual or emotional healing with their herbal work. This can be a wonderful opportunity to help someone embrace traditional healing systems and could be a way to help a person heal even further. When done in the right context, spiritual healing can deepen a person's understanding of their connection with a higher power and can be enlightening. However, there are some concerns about performing spiritual healing ceremonies while someone is still attempting to process a traumatic situation.

Past life regressions, guided shamanic journeys, and other similar meditative events that are designed to help a person transcend space and/or time and discover about their inner self can be extremely disorienting when a person is healing from trauma. If a client is in an early stage of attempting to regulate and integrate their traumatic experience, herbalists who want to utilize such healing rituals would be wise to wait. Waiting can allow you to become more familiar with the client, they can become more comfortable with you, and once that rapport is built they can have a better experience with these traditional healing modalities.

Final thoughts

Retraumatization can shut someone off from your work forever. It can create more issues for them to work through, while also turning them off to natural healing techniques that can be highly effective in the proper setting. We won't always get things right, but working to become more trauma-informed and staying sensitive to our clients' needs is the right place to start.

I've developed a series of small meditations, working up to the full journey that I have used with clients. This can help someone to experience a few minutes of guided meditation while staying in a safe place. If a client wants to try this, it can be a good idea to have quick, five to ten minute guided meditations for them to try. However, do not push someone to do this if they are not ready.

Also, remember that healing is not linear. New events can cause a person's window of tolerance to narrow. Anniversaries of major traumas can cause a person to struggle. Rapport with a person allows them to feel more open to communicating with you. Continuing to pay attention to your regular clients can help you see when they could benefit from going back to more of an extrinsic "cocoon" strategy as we discussed in chapter seven.

Mindfulness and meditation practices are tools that can be used for many people during their healing process. As trauma-informed healers, we must recognize that this is not a one-size-fits-all scenario. Commit to learning and incorporating more options for meditations to support as many clients as possible.

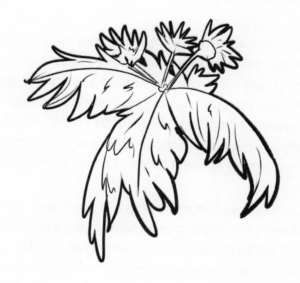

Chapter 14
Yoga and Movement Therapies

I debated whether or not it would be beneficial to add the next three chapters to a book mainly devoted to plant medicine. As herbalists, our main focus is on plants, but our natural tendency to embrace a more holistic approach tends to find us exploring other fields. Many of us branch into therapies such as energy medicine. Frequently, we also find ourselves devoted to teaching different forms of healing movement, such as yoga.

Even without formal training in movement medicine, most herbalists find themselves encouraging lifestyle habit change alongside the plant therapies we know to be beneficial. Drinking more water, practicing better sleep hygiene, and exercise regimens. Because of this, we should be aware of some general considerations when suggesting movement medicine practices.

Movement therapy trauma-informed language considerations

Chapter five is my in-depth discussion on general trauma-informed language for herbalists. There are also some phrases specifically heard in exercise settings that do not fit into a trauma-informed environment. As a yoga teacher, I avoid certain phrasing or suggestions that might cause a person to become activated during class. As you read through this section, take some time to journal other ideas that come to mind.

Bringing someone's attention to certain body parts while they are in a receptive, open mode could activate a response. People who struggle with body dysmorphia, eating disorders, or sexual assault could find themselves facing unwanted memories. I avoid words such as "tummy" or "stomach" in favor of abdomen. I don't use "butt" or "buttocks." I avoid mentioning the inside of the mouth, the teeth, or tongue during yoga nidra scanning.

We should always work to encourage people to listen to their body and explore what feels right. I commonly offer variations of a pose, reminding people to do what feels right today. If you aren't well versed in alternative options for your poses, look to people such as Jivana Heyman, C-IAYT, E-RYT 500. His book, Accessible Yoga: Poses and Practices for Every Body can help shift your paradigm into how to offer other options.

On a similar note, avoid using phrases that rank different alignments as "better" than others. When someone says they are going to demonstrate "the fullest expression of the pose" and then immediately twist into a positioning that a person who has an amputated arm could not perform - they are inadvertently suggesting that person is unable to ever fully experience the healing that a particular movement offers. Other phrasing such as harder or easier, first or second, and beginner or advanced can create a barrier. Adjusting your phrasing to say things like "another option" or "experiment with this..." can help all people feel more connected with the practice you are offering.

The invitation to practice should always feel soft and inviting in a trauma-informed space. Barking commands, pushing people with tough love, and harsh wording can cause a person to spend their energy regulating their trauma response instead of being able to focus on their healing. Recognize that pushing people with unresolved trauma can cause them to begin associating exercise with a feeling of panic.

Trauma, exercise, and panic

Some people who experience trauma may struggle with exercise. During exercise, your heart rate rises, you become flushed, and your breathing intensifies. What else has similar sensations? Anxiety attacks.

If a client tells you they are uncomfortable with exercise because they find it causes them to experience panic, believe them. Encourage them to get cleared by their physician for exercise. Once they are cleared, encourage them to start slow. Extremely slow.

When this happened to me, I could only walk five minutes per day. It took me months to get back to what felt like a normally paced thirty minute walk. Painfully slow progress is common, so do not be surprised if someone takes longer than expected.

Work with your client to determine what type of exercise they prefer. If it is yoga, look into different types and intensity levels of classes offered in your area. Some people start with restorative yoga and work their way up to yin, maybe trying some chair yoga, then gentle, then perhaps a vinyasa flow. The key is to continue making tiny improvements when possible.

Yoga poses that could activate trauma responses

One of my teachers, Michelle Young C-IAYT, E-RYT 500, discusses several yoga poses that you should consider because they can leave a person feeling vulnerable. Exposed positions can activate a traumatic response in students with unresolved trauma. These poses include down dog, standing forward fold, happy baby, thread the needle, cat/cow, and reclined bound angle pose.

I debate whether we should blacklist these poses and call them "poses to avoid". In some situations, some of these poses could be healing. There are also ways to modify several of these poses to feel less vulnerable. It's possible to physically modify them, but there are more philosophically based modification options as well.

One of my colleagues, Nancy Cunningham, E-RYT 500, YACEP emphasizes the idea that understanding the history and mythology behind poses can help us find unique modifications. We may find it is best to offer alternatives to these poses that have similar benefits. When appropriate, we can also offer the stories and discussion aspects during class to help our students further.

Yoga poses that can reduce trauma responses

Many poses can be helpful at encouraging regulation and reducing trauma responses. As with everything we discuss in this book, each person is different and these ideas might work better during certain parts of their healing journey. Always continue to learn and adjust ideas according to what works best for each of your clients.

Forward folds help tone the vagus nerve and activate the ventral vagal response. This helps us feel calm and more present in the moment. While a standing forward fold might cause someone to feel vulnerable, seated forward folds are usually well received. I start many of my trauma-informed classes with a forward fold and sometimes return to this forward fold if I see students' body language shift into a more alert state.

Yoga flows that do a lot of poses requiring you to alternate sides can create a gentle bi-lateral stimulation in your brain. This could possibly create better communication in the brain and might make it easier for a person to feel connected to their body during class. Bi-lateral stimulation is similar to the practices that are utilized for EMDR therapy. I love to implement several poses that cause us to switch sides and do the same pose on the opposite side, such as Warrior II or Tree pose.

In her book Relax and Renew, Judith Lasater, PhD, PT suggested that moving the spine in all directions can have a calming effect. While she was discussing this in the context of restorative yoga, I have experimented with using a similar philosophy in trauma-informed classes. It does appear that offering a flow that allows the spine to gently twist and bend can help many people who are struggling with regulation.

Grounding postures connect us to the Earth and help us feel the resonance she provides. I find many poses can be considered grounding, if the right cues are offered. "Feel your connection through your feet" or "ground down with your hands to feel the resonance of the Earth" are two examples of cues that could encourage students to ground.

Chest openers are great in some situations, but can be activating in others. Think about a person who is in the habit of hunching over in the face of stress. It is almost as if they're attempting to protect their heart center. Chest openers invite us to open that heart center back up; we stand strong in the vulnerability of that openness. In a trauma-informed class, I will make a point to encourage students to play with how different amounts of stretch may emotionally feel different. I like to follow a chest opener with a forward fold or grounding posture.

Hip openers are another set of postures that are good under the right circumstances. They can feel vulnerable to some, but can also help to release a lot of emotion. Similar to chest openers, I encourage students to be aware of the emotions that come up as they adjust their alignment and change the stretch.

Physical touch for adjustments

I choose to keep physical adjustments to a minimum when I teach yoga classes. I rarely find I need to touch a student in order to help them adjust. There are usually ways to phrase an adjustment or give a visual cue that will suffice. But what happens when we genuinely find students might benefit from an adjustment?

When discussing muscle testing assessment tools in chapter nine, I mention having clients opt in. This same theory applies for physical touch. Instead of announcing at the beginning of class: "if you don't want to be touched for adjustments, please let me know" (opt out protocol), consider saying this: "if you believe that it could be helpful for me to physically adjust you during class, please let me know" (opt in protocol).

When opt out protocols have been used, a person may worry they don't know what is best for them. They may choose to defer to your judgment, knowing that the physical touch could be jarring for them. They may even spend class worrying about the possibility of being physically touched at a moment in which they're vulnerable and open in practice.

In an opt in protocol setting, a person has more autonomy. You are offering an option, but not indicating that the physical adjustment would be considered the norm. The people who want that type of support can speak up and others are able to focus on practice without worry.

Pranayama

As discussed in the last chapter, focusing on breathing can be a difficult task for certain people with unresolved trauma. So how do we approach pranayama in a way that supports everyone? As with many of the modalities we've discussed, my answer to this depends on the situation. Take my thoughts, consider them as you prepare your next trauma-informed offerings, and come up with a solution that works best for the people you are working with.

One option may be to offer two different trauma-informed practices each week. One could have pranayama and the other one does not have any breathwork related practices. Advertise accordingly and people will be able to choose which of the two works best for them.

Another option may be to offer two different practices during breathwork. One of the practices is directly related to breathwork. The other practice could be available for people who are interested in focusing on another anchor, such as the music or the physical sensation of their fingers touching their thumb.

Alternate nostril breathing, or nadi shodhana, is a practice in which you inhale through one nostril and exhale through the other. Then you reverse: inhale through the second nostril, exhaling through the first. This breath technique causes a person to focus on one side of the face, then the other. This could be helpful for students with unresolved trauma that respond well to bi-lateral stimulation.

Alternate nostril breathing can be performed as a visualization with similar benefits. Instead of putting your fingers in front of your nose, poised to close the nostril not in use, you just imagine focusing the air into the appropriate nostril. I like to utilize the visualization technique for myself when I am feeling overwhelmed and want a quick, recentering breath. I see this used sometimes during Yoga Nidra or other situations where the goal is to reduce physical movement.

Yoga nidra

Yoga nidra, or the yoga of sleep, is a meditative form of yoga that traditionally consists of a person lying very still. The teacher then moves them through their subtle energetic bodies with guided meditation. This is a powerful meditation technique that can help a person rewire portions of their brain to be more responsive and mindful.

Dr. Richard Miller has studied the ability of yoga nidra to support patients with PTSD. He has a patented system of meditation called iRest yoga nidra. Because of his research using his iRest yoga nidra techniques, more groups are beginning to recognize the efficacy of treating trauma through yoga nidra practices.

However, this does not mean yoga nidra is a cure all for every person struggling with unresolved trauma. Traditional yoga nidra practices may or may not work well for an individual, and you as a trauma-informed teacher must consider what aspects of yoga nidra may need to be adjusted for your students. There are several things to consider when offering a trauma-informed yoga nidra session.

I like to let the class know up front what we will be doing throughout the session. I will briefly mention what each section is going to offer, in order to reduce any sensation of anxiousness of the unknown. I will also mention if there are alternative practices that can be done in a section that might be activating to someone. Especially for sections of the practice such as body scanning.

Body scanning, which is a central aspect of yoga nidra, may be uncomfortable for some people. Bringing total awareness to each body part may be difficult for some. If a student mentions this, you can invite them to utilize a different practice during this time. They may also decide that yoga nidra isn't the best fit for them at this moment, so you can help them choose another path.

Body scanning guidance is traditionally done by starting at one hand, flowing up the arm, and following a path all over the body. One trauma-informed version of body scanning that I love to use is to jump from one side to the other.

"Right hand"

"Left hand"

"Right wrist"

"Left wrist"

And so on.

This can allow for a bi-lateral stimulation effect during the initial phases of yoga nidra. Many of my students have found this version a bit more difficult to keep up with at first. However, once they get accustomed to the flow they find it is beneficial.

In a trauma-informed yoga nidra class, I will offer for people to remain in a seated position, or use any number of restorative poses that may feel good to them. A reclining restorative pose can allow a person to receive the same kind of deep physical relaxation without feeling completely vulnerable on their back. I will also mention that if something becomes activating that they can sit up and open their eyes, staying on their mat until practice is ended.

I always request that students stay on their mat for the duration of yoga nidra. This is because it can be activating for other students if a person begins walking around the space in the midst of such a deep, meditative practice. The low light combined with the vulnerable mental state can cause this type of disturbance to be particularly jarring.

Some yoga nidra techniques encourage guided visualizations. I do not include many guided visualizations when working with a general public trauma-informed yoga nidra class. We cannot know what might activate a bad memory for someone in a general class. While many of us consider the beach a relaxing environment, there may be someone in the class who experienced a terrifying situation on a beach.

If I have a group that has worked with me for a while in a semi-private setting, or I am with someone one on one, I can usually craft a visualization set that will not create a traumatic memory activation. You may find you like to work with visualization options for these clients. However, you can also encourage visualization and mindful observation of whatever a student is seeing in their minds eye without giving guiding prompts.

Because of the research that has been done showing yoga nidra as a well tolerated option for many people, students may come to class believing that yoga nidra is perfect for everyone. Similar to the mindfulness meditation we discussed in the last chapter, they may be disoriented if they have a bad experience. If a student mentions they are struggling, always validate their feelings. Then help them determine what might be a better support option at this time.

Somatic experiencing

Dr. Peter Levine has pioneered work in the field of somatic experiencing. There are many aspects of his work that might be applied in a yoga setting. The ideas he discusses regarding how the body physically holds trauma can be seen in the way people struggle with certain poses, how other poses may release emotions, and how people respond to different movements in general.

Somatic yoga is an umbrella term that is used to indicate practices that help a person to feel more grounded in their body. These practices can assist a person with feeling more secure in their mind-body connection. Two of the aspects of Dr. Levine's teaching that I see utilized in somatic yoga settings are titration and pendulation.

Titration is the process of noticing a sensation that is at the edge of the comfort zone and sitting with it. You aren't trying to push, just being aware of that stretch. In these moments of noticing, we choose not to judge the sensation. We aren't afraid of it, we aren't attempting to embody it. We are just allowing it to be in the moment.

Pendulation is swinging back and forth. We may spend time noticing a small, uncomfortable sensation. But then we activate a resource that helps us go back to a place where we feel calm and supported.

It is important to note that titration and pendulation are only beneficial if a person is already feeling safe enough to start healing. The safety we provide as practitioners allows a person to move into a place where they can process different physical sensations that indicate trauma that has become trapped in the body.

If somatic experiencing interests you, there are many trainings that can support your journey to learn more. This brief description is not enough knowledge to safely use these techniques with someone who is recovering from unresolved trauma. You can begin by looking at one of Dr. Levine's books. While Waking the Tiger is a classic, I have really enjoyed the updated information he provides in his book In an Unspoken Voice.

Mantras

After working with some of the somatic experiencing ideas Dr. Levine teaches, I stumbled upon his "voo" technique. This consists of intoning the word "voo" on a long exhale, in an almost mantra-like action. He suggests that his "voo" technique is similar to chants and mantras that are found throughout many practices. As yoga teachers, we have access to many mantras that could be helpful for our clients.

There may be some vagus nerve toning that occurs with mantras. It could be the deeper breaths and diaphragmatic breathing working toward relaxation. It might be the breath acting as an anchoring point that works similar to other mindfulness anchors. You might feel more connected and grounded while using mantras that you intentionally chose. Whatever the mechanism, mantra work can be very useful for people who are working through trauma.

The bija or seed mantras are one syllable mantras with a similar feel to the "voo" technique that Dr. Levine suggests. Learning these sounds and their meanings can be a helpful tool. There are several seed mantras with important significance.

The bija mantras that are connected to the seven chakras may be a beneficial starting place for you to work with intoning. These may be helpful in your own practice, but you may also find they are beneficial in group settings. The seven mantras I use are Lam (root), Vam (sacral), Ram (solar plexus), Yam (heart), Ham (throat), Om (third eye), and silence for the crown chakra.

Final thoughts

While my focus in this chapter has been on yoga, there are many other movement therapies that you may choose to utilize. Pilates can have similar benefits on the nervous system. Forest bathing on nature hikes can have emotional and physical benefits.

Tai chi and Qigong have synchronized movement in a group setting, which is a fantastic way to start rewiring one's brain for connection. They also have energy healing aspects that can support a person on a subtle energy level. One of my early experiences with energy work was through Ki gong, a similar movement therapy utilized in Tang Soo Do martial arts. In the next chapter, we will dive more into vibrational healing techniques such as Reiki and chakra balancing.

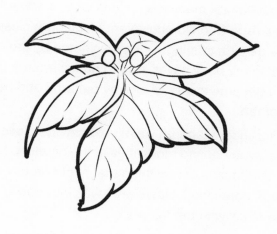

Chapter 15
Reiki and Energy Medicine

Energy medicine is my first love. I grew up around several herbalists and saw the benefits of plants, but I really fell in love with natural medicine options when I started taking Ki Gong (the Tang Soo Do equivalent of Qigong) classes as part of my martial arts training. I was fascinated by the changes I could feel in my body. I was able to notice energy shifts before I got sick. I became aware of energy patterns and began noticing them in others.

Florence, Alabama wasn't exactly the place for learning "new age" type healing modalities in the nineties. My Ki Gong teacher didn't focus on anything that might be too woo-woo for the general population. However, I was introduced to concepts that have stuck with me for years.

We were taught to listen to our bodies and notice the flow of energy. I could tell when I was getting sick by the way my energy flow would "reverse". Fellow students caught their own illnesses well before other methods would have been useful. Was this just a matter of slowing down and noticing our bodies? Or was there a subtle life force shift detected?

I did not spend much time wondering about whether or not this was mindful attention or something more esoteric. At thirteen I had a thousand extra curricular activities and didn't have time to wonder about the mysteries of the universe. But as I got older and discovered Reiki, I began to suspect there was something more to energy work than mindful attention alone.

Energy medicine works hand in hand with herbalism. I have already discussed the pinnacle of this combination: flower essences. This chapter is designed to discuss a bit about energy work that could be applied alongside herbal remedies.

Herbalism and energy

Many healing systems describe some form of vital life force, qi, prana, or resonance. All of these different names indicate the subtle energy flow that all living things possess. Most of these systems acknowledge the ability of herbs to rebalance these subtle energies. Honoring the place of herbs in energy work can help us to create a positive experience for clients.

For instance, I once had a client that visited me who was suffering from severe panic attacks. The doctors could not determine what was happening to cause the attacks. After a bit of discussion, I found out she was using (*way* too much) cinnamon in an attempt to support healthy blood sugar. With her natural tendency toward heat, it became obvious that the cinnamon was overstimulating and creating a sensation of panic. We adjusted accordingly, added some cooling stevia to her protocol, and the panic subsided.

Traditional Chinese Medicine, Ayurveda, and Western Herbalism all have some form of subtle energetics that can help create balance in the body. But our subtle life force energy can bring healing from other angles as well. Herbalists can utilize healing energy in many situations without ever learning energy healing modalities.

Conscientiously harvesting herbs so that vital energy is preserved is one way energy healing comes into play for herbalists. Many herbalists practice requesting permission from plants to harvest. Part of the requesting permission can be telling the plants about why you are harvesting them. Tell them about the people they are helping. Create that connection and strengthen intention.

You may find harvesting at certain times of the lunar cycle creates a different feel to the herbs you use. Harvesting at the new moon brings energies that may invite a person to look inward and become more self aware. Harvesting during the waxing moon has a build up of energy that can be helpful for someone who is fatigued. Harvesting at the full moon creates a feel of manifestation. The waxing moon energies help someone to release that which no longer serves them.

Another practice many herbalists use is infusing extractions with healing energy. Just holding a tincture or a salve after completion and charging it with loving vibes can create another dimension of healing activation. Many of these energy healing options tend to be well tolerated, though on occasion I have had clients struggle with energy work.

Trauma and energy work

Unresolved trauma may make it difficult for someone to feel comfortable with energy healing. Energy healing tends to open a person up and it can cause someone to feel vulnerable. Many of my clients start with other modalities and we work up to energy work.

I personally have had two clients that initially claimed that Reiki energy made them feel worse. Both were struggling with complex trauma. They both told me that the times they had tried Reiki in the past it had made them sick to their stomach afterward.

Before working with me, there were several one-off failed attempts at using Reiki as a healing energy. The first time one of them mentioned it, I thought maybe it was just a mental block. By the time the second client had told me about it, I realized there was something more going on.

After several sessions and careful introduction of Reiki, they both came to love energy work. This has caused me to feel that the main issue wasn't the Reiki - it was that they didn't feel safe with the other healers before being put in a vulnerable place. This wasn't necessarily the fault of the other healers, but if they had been trauma-informed my clients might have found relief sooner.

When someone comes to me and they declare Reiki a bad fit, I never press them to try it. I want to work with them on more tangible, physical solutions first. Once they develop a sense of safety, we will revisit the option. However, Reiki can be a powerful tool when someone is comfortable with it!

Breakthroughs

For many, Reiki is a powerful tool that encourages healing progress. Quiet time on the Reiki table can allow for your clients to slow down and focus their attention on their needs. If we create a safe space, our clients can experience a ventral vagal state while the energy is working on a subtle level. In this state, they are able to come into a place of clarity that allows for good decisions to be made and emotional healing to occur.

I've watched people have amazing breakthrough moments on my table. For instance, Kayla had been coming to me for support for a few months. We had been doing some energy work almost every session. One day, we did Reiki and chakra balancing for almost an entire hour.

After the session ended, she sat up rather quickly. She did not say much and seemed ready to head out the door before I was finished giving her recommendations. After we got through, she left and I wondered if the session had really been what she needed.

The next time we got together, Kayla told me about what she had experienced at our previous session. She said she had become very calm and started thinking about a visualization her therapist had been trying to use with her. She had struggled through several therapy sessions, unable to complete this visualization.

However, during our energy healing session she was able to complete her visualization and had a breakthrough. She had been so excited that she could hardly wait to call her therapist. She was thrilled that she had made that progress.

I never even knew what the visualization was. I do not think Kayla ever told me the subject matter of her breakthrough. There was no discussion prior to our session about those topics. This was all done because she was able to get comfortable and focus on her healing during her energy session. I believe the Reiki helped to open her up and inspired her to revisit the visualization exercise while in a ventral vagal state.

Reiki

Usui Reiki is a simple system to learn and a tough system to master. Each level comes with attunements, which help us to tap into the specific frequencies needed for healing. There are also symbols that are revealed at different points during the training process. During Reiki healing, the practitioner acts as a conduit, allowing the Reiki energy to flow and direct the healing process.

Tradition holds that Dr. Mikao Usui was given the healing system of Reiki after a 21 day fast on Mount Kurama. He went on to teach over 2,000 students. One of those students, Chujiro Hayashi, taught Hawayo Takata. Madame Takata is responsible for bringing Reiki to America and helping to establish the healing system in the West.

Reiki has the potential to relieve many uncomfortable symptoms. One study even shows that Reiki was better than massage therapy at relieving fatigue and anxiety[1]. It's a relatively simple system to implement with very few contraindications.

As Usui Reiki has become popular, other forms of healing that require attunements have been presented. Many of these healing arts utilize "reiki" in their name, even if they are not from the original Usui system. Crystal reiki, gold reiki, holy fire reiki... There are so many different forms of reiki that are available for you to consider.

While many people lay flat on the Reiki table, my trauma-informed offerings include the ability to sit up and even participate in quiet activity. I have one client who brings her crochet and works on her latest project. Another client prefers to read.

On occasion, I find it helpful to include my client in the conscious energy healing process. The sessions run a bit different, but may be better tolerated by some. Instead of my client lying quietly and enjoying the relaxation, I communicate with them to steer the session. Although many people come to my table and enjoy the chance to completely melt into the silence, some find the interaction helpful to keep themselves grounded.

While Reiki itself isn't very interactive, there are other energy healing techniques that can be utilized. I find there are easy correlations with the chakras that can be quickly implemented in sessions. When a client decides an interactive session is best, I tend to turn toward chakra balancing for best results.

The chakras

The seven main chakras are a recurring theme in my work as a trauma-informed herbalist. In chapter ten, we discussed the association between certain essential oil scents and the chakras. In the next chapter, we will revisit the chakra centers in the context of sound healing and the notes of the C-scale. These associations are helpful in creating balance through different methods. Anodea Judith's book, Eastern Body,

Western Mind, shows fascinating correspondences between each chakra and psychological aspects.

There is a relationship between our energetic bodies and the psychological outcome of our experiences. The chakras can be affected by traumatic events and we may be more susceptible to experiencing unresolved trauma if a chakra is unbalanced. I consider chakra balancing a great complementary therapy to use when someone is first starting work with their therapist to tackle significant trauma responses. It was a lifesaver for me when I first went through EMDR (eye movement desensitization and reprocessing) for my PTSD.

There are many ways to approach chakra healing. You may choose to encourage clients to explore the use of color. Some people may be more drawn to the connections of certain stones and crystals. Herbs can also be a beneficial energetic support for different chakra centers. Try different ways to rebalance your chakra centers and see what you connect with the most.

Muladhara

The root chakra, muladhara, is strongly correlated with our fight or flight response. When the adrenals are oversensitive from too much stress, nourishing the root chakra can help to encourage their healing. Fear and its descendents are commonly linked to the root chakra.

The initial development of the root chakra happens very early in our life. Within the first couple of years of life, the root chakra is fully formed and supporting the body. Healthy development gives a person a sense of stability and ease. Traumas relating to experiences in the womb, birth, and the first few months of life can arrest the development of the root chakra.

All traumas have a tendency to impact the root chakra because of its correlation with the adrenals and with feeling safe. Any trauma where a person is stuck may create a significant impact in the root energy. Traumas where someone loses their home or livelihood are especially damaging to the root chakra.

Shane had lost their father and was struggling with an almost simultaneous job loss. They found themselves swirling in the sensation of their trauma experiences, like a leaf in a whirlpool. The gravity that was holding them to this Earth was gone. Instead, they described how the magnetic pull of the trauma was keeping them together.

This pull had them re-living their trauma with anyone that would listen. The constant retraumatization was making it harder and harder to move forward with life. While Shane had multiple imbalances, the root chakra re-balancing was the most important aspect of their recovery. Without the root chakra work we did together, they would not have been able to find an anchor to pull them away from the trauma.

A lack of strong boundaries may develop from certain traumatic situations, indicating a need to nourish the root chakra. Feelings such as never having enough to be safe, feeling the need to try to plan for all possibilities, and being unable to connect with the earth are signs of root chakra imbalance. Depending on how a person responds to their experiences, they may find themselves feeling floaty and disconnected or they may be so grounded that movement feels uncomfortable.

The color red is associated with the root chakra. Stones with red in them such as red jasper and bloodstone are commonly used to heal the root chakra. Grounding, dark colored stones are also used. Think of things like hematite or black obsidian. I recommend making waist beads with these stones, as wearing them close to the chakra is beneficial.

Any physical movement that encourages a connection with the body can be beneficial to someone who is struggling with a root chakra connection. Yoga practices that focus on mindful movement are wonderful. Powerful poses that encourage a sense of strength and connection to the Earth are also useful.

Grounding exercises are nourishing to the root chakra. This can be as simple as exhaling and feeling your energy seep into the ground. Walking barefoot outside for a few minutes can strengthen our feeling of being grounded. Even just being seated outside, with the intention of connecting to the sounds of nature around you can be a grounding experience.

Any herbs that create a sense of grounding will benefit the root chakra. Ashwagandha (*Withania somnifera*), chicory (*Cichorium intybus*), blackberry (*Rubus fruticosus*), and eleuthero (*Eleutherococcus senticosus*) are all medicinal herbs I find useful. In general, root herbs have a strong connection with the root chakra.

Svadhisthana

The sacral chakra, svadhisthana, is connected to our creativity and sexual energy. Anytime this center is off, we may find it difficult to produce creative results. Writer's block is one of the more obvious creative interferences that can occur when the sacral chakra is imbalanced. Someone who is struggling with romantic relationships may also find their sacral chakra needs nourishment.

The sacral chakra's main development starts when we are a few months old and lasts until we are a toddler. Any trauma that is experienced during this time frame can interfere with our creativity or sense of healthy sexual relationships later in life. A client may find themselves constantly starting creative projects, but moving on to the next "shiny" thing before they complete the first project. Someone who is struggling with sacral chakra imbalance may also exhibit addictive behavior or a general attitude of being unsatisfied with their physical experience.

Sexual trauma is recognized as one of the main types of trauma that can create imbalances in the sacral chakra. Other traumas around infertility, miscarriage, and womb connections to our family can affect the health of the sacral chakra. Trauma involving our creative pursuits can also cause the sacral chakra to suffer.

Healing can be activated in svadhisthana with gold and orange colors. Crystals such as carnelian, amber, and sunstone can nourish this creative center. I love to use yellow gold jewelry when I am trying to build resonance in the sacral chakra.

Trying new creative endeavors can help rebuild a healthy sacral chakra. Take that creative writing class or sign up for the ballroom dance course. It's not about becoming a professional; it's about embracing creativity as a form of pleasure.

Gardening is another activity that can create a stronger sacral chakra. Participating in the creation of something that can bring pleasure to the sense of taste is nourishing the sacral chakra energy on many levels. I encourage you to plant herbs or veggies that grow well in your region and that you enjoy eating.

Herbaceous plants that are commonly used as spices are associated with the sacral chakra. Rosemary (*Salvia rosmarinus*), sage (*Salvia officinalis*), oregano (*Origanum vulgare*), and thyme (*Thymus vulgaris*) are all herbaceous plants. Using any form of spice on your food helps support a strong sacral chakra energy.

Manipura

The solar plexus chakra, manipura, is connected to our sense of self and our ability to transform. Digestive processes, the transformation of physical food into energy, is ruled by the solar plexus. Our willpower is closely linked with solar plexus energy. Subtle emotional processes are also governed by manipura. Think of things like transmuting anger into productivity or grief into an urge to help others.

The solar plexus' initial development occurs between eighteen months and about five years old. At this age, children begin to notice their sense of self. They may want to be more independent and may begin to exercise their will. There is nothing more willful than a toddler who has discovered the word "no".

Any trauma that damages our sense of self can affect the solar plexus chakra. Commonly, people with PTSD report struggling with their sense of self and its link to their trauma experience[2]. These self identity struggles somatically manifest as digestive issues for many people.

Chronic traumas can also affect the solar plexus chakra. If a person begins to feel that they cannot escape a traumatic situation, they may begin to doubt their transformational power. Manipura is affected when a person begins to feel they have no capability to change their situation.

The islets of Langerhans, the cells in the pancreas that secrete insulin and glucagon, are associated with the solar plexus chakra energy. When someone shows signs of insulin resistance after a traumatic event, I encourage them to support the solar plexus. Because energetic work can be done alongside almost any conventional treatment plan, I feel this is a safe option for most people who are struggling with digestion-related disease.

Digestive issues are common with high stress levels. Many aspects of the stomach and intestines can be affected. The information that is coming out around the gut microbiome and its importance in mental health is fascinating. Since the solar plexus is so closely linked with gut health, I like to nurture this subtle energy any time someone is struggling with digestive issues.

Yellow is the color most frequently associated with the solar plexus. Citrine, tiger's eye, and yellow jasper are stones that are employed to support healthy solar plexus energy. Goldstone is a manmade stone that I have found to also have beneficial healing effects on the solar plexus.

Any activity that consists of purposeful transmutation will help to strengthen the solar plexus chakra. There are many ways to purposefully shift the energy around us. Changing our perception about an event over which we have no control is one form of transmutation.

Choosing to let go of harmful self perceptions is another. I like to incorporate the element of fire into this practice, since fire is strongly associated with the solar plexus. Writing a few things that I'm ready to release on a piece of paper and then intentionally (and safely!) burning it has a very cathartic effect.

Trees and woodsy type plants are associated with the solar plexus chakra. Willow (*Salix alba*), white oak (*Quercus alba*), and cascara sagrada (*Frangula purshiana*) are examples of these bark elements that can be useful for the solar plexus. You can also associate any herb that supports healthy upper digestion with the solar plexus. Liver support herbs, carminatives, and even prebiotic rich plants could be considered associated with manipura.

Anahata

The heart chakra, anahata, is the seat of unconditional love, healthy relationships, and healing. Boundaries with others may be difficult if the heart chakra is imbalanced. It is also associated with the thymus gland, so there are implications for the immune system as well.

Developmental activation in the heart chakra starts around age four and continues until we are seven or eight years old. This is the prime stage for a person to determine how they belong: with friends, in a family unit, and in the bigger picture. The consistent yin and yang, give and take of relationships is first experienced in this development stage.

Relationship related traumas can directly affect the heart chakra. Domestic violence, intimate partner violence, and other relationship abuses can cause a person to need more nourishment in their heart chakra. After such events, boundaries with relationships and trusting people in general can be difficult.

Stress affects the immune system's ability to function. When someone goes through any sort of traumatic event, they may find their immune system weakened or frazzled. Frequent low grade infections, feeling run down, and odd autoimmune symptoms can crop up after trauma. Nourishing the heart center as part of a complementary immune support response can help.

Traumas that stem from chronic illness can wear on the heart chakra energy. People who are struggling with chronic illness may feel isolated from their friends and may feel they are a burden on their caretakers. Chronic illnesses can also strain the immune system. Since there are aspects on both the physical and emotional front that are affected, someone who has a chronic illness will benefit from nourishing anahata.

Green and pink colors are associated with heart chakra energies. Stones such as malachite, aventurine, unakite, and rose quartz are used for heart chakra healing. Wearing a longer necklace that features one or more of these stones can be beneficial.

Activities that encourage connection with others are helpful for the heart chakra. Volunteering in a capacity that feels safe and comfortable can make a difference in anahata's energy. We may normally think of big gestures as necessary for a healing effect, but that is not the case.

After COVID, I suffered from significant fatigue. I wanted to immediately go to the scene and offer healing support after a shooting occurred at a church here in Birmingham, but I could not leave the house. The only thing I could do was send tea and crochet prayer shawls for others. If all you can do is a small, quiet gesture, do it with all your might. Not only will you still gain a sense of connectedness, you will bring joy to someone else who might be struggling.

Connection to humans is vital, but supporting heart energy through the connection to nature is also important for someone's trauma recovery. Forest bathing, or intentionally spending time surrounded by nature, to regain a sense of well being can even support lower blood pressure$_3$. Plant connections, like those discussed in chapter twelve, can help a person to coregulate and nurture the heart chakra.

Warming herbs that are commonly used in baking are associated with the heart chakra. Think star anise (*Illicium verum*), cinnamon (*Cinnamomum verum*), and clove (*Syzygium aromaticum*). Spicy chai teas can also be a quick way to warm the heart center. These heart chakra herbs always make me think of creating rituals with friends that foster safe connection through unconditional love.

Vishuddha

The throat chakra, vishuddha, governs the energy of speech and being able to communicate ideas to others. This energy is about our capacity to be heard and feel noticed. Women in particular may find their throat chakra energy suppressed, but anyone who has struggled with trauma can be subjected to this imbalance.

Vishuddha begins to develop during the prepubescent time. It can start as early as age seven and continues until age twelve. Any event that happens during this time or revolves around the throat can add to a weakened throat energy.

An interesting note: vishuddha is related to the thyroid gland. Many of my clients come to me with thyroid related issues. Breathing obstructions may also cause throat energy disruption.

Traumas where someone has been choked can cause the throat chakra to be imbalanced. More frequently, I have clients who have felt their voice has been trampled. They may become extremely vocal and loud, as if they're shouting to make sure everyone hears them. The other common response is to become extremely reserved, as if they no longer want to be heard. Many marginalized groups are in need of throat chakra support.

Experiencing systematic discrimination, gaslighting, and dehumanization can all lead to a weakened throat chakra. Any trauma that leaves a person feeling unheard is going to affect vishuddha. We can collectively start the process of healing by actively listening to each other and helping each other to feel heard.

Vishuddha is associated with lighter blue colors. Turquoise and blue lapis are commonly used in throat chakra healing. Blue sandstone is a manmade crystal that can encourage confidence and healing. Using these stones in earrings or a choker type necklace can be a beneficial way to get the support of their healing energies.

Singing, writing, and mantras can be very supportive of the throat chakra. Find time to sing a favorite song to your plants each day to incorporate the plant connection alongside throat chakra healing. Write a heartfelt note to someone to express friendship. Choose a mantra that activates the chakras and get the benefits of ventral vagal toning alongside throat chakra healing.

Minty herbs are nourishing to the throat chakra. Think of a tea that would soothe a sore throat. Peppermint (*Mentha x piperita*), spearmint (*Mentha spicata*), and fennel (*Foeniculum vulgare*) have these qualities. I love to create a cold infusion out of peppermint and a mucilaginous herb such as marshmallow root (*Althaea officinalis*) to coat the throat in a protective, cooling layer.

Ajna

The third eye chakra, ajna, is the intuitive center of the chakra system. Seeing, understanding, and translating your higher purpose into something actionable are actions that stem from the third eye chakra. Visualization of future goals is also ruled by the third eye center.

Many people turn to ajna to focus on metaphysical, superhuman intuition development. I am fascinated by the idea of remote viewing and event prediction, but this isn't the place for a Men Who Stare at Goats-style debate. When someone is struggling with unresolved trauma, nurturing the third eye chakra can help them reorient and see things with clarity.

While the throat chakra governs the communication we offer, ajna governs how we perceive communication we receive. When someone speaks to you, how clearly you interpret the meaning of their communication is based on how strong your third eye chakra is. Trauma affects this perception and can leave someone disoriented. This makes it harder for a person to comfortably re-connect with others.

As we get older, we rise further into the more ethereal energies. The teenage years rule the development of ajna. The first awareness of collective unconsciousness can be detected during this phase. Becoming more in tune with the intuitive sense and being able to use real world experience to recognize when something is working or not is part of ajna development.

Trauma that causes a person to question their decision making skills affects the third eye chakra. Anything that causes a person to second guess their intuition and natural radar is going to weaken the third eye. This could be a situation where someone else has emotionally abused them and now they are unsure of their ability to make good choices.

This could also be a situation where someone made a benign decision that precipitated a traumatic event. For instance, one of my clients suffered significant guilt around their decision to drive to a different store than usual. A car wreck occurred, seriously injuring their friend. They felt that the event was their fault because they decided to go across town to a different place than they usually went.

While there are many aspects of this situation that a cognitive behavioral therapist was able to help my client work through, there was also a need for complementary support. Before we started using third eye chakra healing techniques, he was stuck in the therapy sessions. Once we did a few weeks of energy healing, he was able to move forward and resolve the feelings of guilt. His therapist helped him to process the feelings and begin trusting his intuition once more, but the energy healing was an important part of his healing process.

Dark blues and indigo are associated with the third eye chakra. Sodalite and labradorite are commonly used. I also love clear quartz, to help bring clarity to the intuitive senses. Fluorite is another I find myself drawn to, as it helps facilitate the communication between the throat, third eye, and crown chakras.

People with unresolved trauma can benefit from activities such as keeping a note of intuitive nudges that they had during the day that produce a positive outcome. Notice when acquiescing to these moments of intuition brings about extra blessings. This can be especially helpful when it causes you to notice being in tune with another person.

Some of the herbs that are associated with the third eye chakra have fruity tastes. Rose hips (*Rosa canina*), hibiscus (*Hibiscus sabdariffa*), and lemon balm (*Melissa officinalis*) are fantastic options. These teas can be helpful for almost anyone needing third eye support.

Other herbs that are known to help open up intuition are also regularly recommended for third eye support. For someone who is still dealing with unresolved trauma, the untethering effects of these herbs could be unsettling. Many of these herbs can also interfere with psychotropic medications. For trauma-informed care, I tend to stay away from the intuition herbs and focus on herbs with the fruity tastes.

Sahasrara

The crown chakra, sahasrara, is our connection to the spiritual realm and to the higher self. Transcendence and self actualization is realized when the crown chakra is strong. A sense of self examination and empathy is also connected to the crown chakra

Sahasrara's main development occurs once a person begins reaching adulthood. The beginning of our search for meaning creates a strong activation in the crown chakra. We continue to filter our experiences through the crown chakra to update our sense of purpose in this physical world.

Philosophy, religion, and spiritual practices are commonly associated with the crown chakra. Religious trauma can affect our connection to spiritual things. When someone has been harmed by organized religion, their crown chakra can become weakened.

Curiosity and a natural thirst for knowledge is also associated with a healthy crown chakra. When someone has struggled with unresolved trauma, they may no longer be inclined to explore things that interest them. Instead of looking to learn new things, they are stuck in the same daily routine. Healing in the crown chakra can help to reignite that spark of intellectual interest.

Purple, gold, silver, white, and opalescence are all colors that have been associated with the crown chakra. Amethyst, tanzanite, charoite, and opalite can be balancing to the crown chakra. Selenite is another stone that is used in a wand form for healing that can be helpful.

Meditation is a wonderful tool to connect further to the crown chakra. If someone is not far enough along in their healing journey to benefit from meditation, walking a labyrinth can have similar benefits on sahasrara. Almost any quiet, contemplative activity will have nurturing effects on the crown energies.

Floral herbs are associated with the crown chakra. Jasmine (*Jasminum grandiflorum*), lavender (*Lavandula angustifolia*), and honeysuckle (*Lonicera caprifolium*) are all nurturing to sahasrara. I love making a floral based tea before walking the labyrinth to help me open that connection.

Trauma-informed energy work

I will never forget one of the first times I had a person struggle severely during a Reiki session. She dissociated and had a hard time coming back at the end of the session. It was scary - even though we did a lot of grounding exercises, she left relatively present in her body, and followed up promptly with her therapist.

This incident was one of the things that initiated my interest in what we could do to make energy healing and meditation more trauma sensitive. I had seen clients make breakthroughs in energy sessions that they had been working to achieve with their therapists for months. I knew that energy work could be helpful. I needed to understand how to set an environment in which it could be most supportive.

Safety is the number one concern. As I mentioned at the beginning of this chapter, it can be difficult for people to dive straight into an energy session if they do not feel safe. Having tangible activities for someone to focus on can sometimes help a person find that sense of safety during a session.

Tangible activities can be as simple as a fidget tool. I love offering adult coloring books as a mindfulness practice during sessions. Clients who want to read or do other quiet activities are welcome to do so.

Mentioning these things ahead of time can help your initial sessions go smoothly with clients. I let people know about the trauma-informed options ahead of their first session. You may choose to mention your accommodations on your website or other materials. Communicating the options you offer could help someone with unresolved trauma come to see you - they might have otherwise shied away from the thought of having to lie still for an hour.

Energy work is a wonderful way to work with people who have unresolved trauma. If you can adjust your practice to be more inclusive, more people will find the benefits. Vibrational medicine is a powerful tool for healing, and trauma-informed herbalists can incorporate its healing power into their work. In the next chapter, we talk more about vibrational medicine from the angle of sound therapy.

References

1. Vergo, M. T., Pinkson, B. M., Broglio, K., Li, Z., & Tosteson, T. D. (2018). Immediate Symptom Relief After a First Session of Massage Therapy or Reiki in Hospitalized Patients: A 5-Year Clinical Experience from a Rural Academic Medical Center. *Journal of alternative and complementary medicine (New York, N.Y.)*, 24(8), 801–808. https://doi.org/10.1089/acm.2017.0409

2. Lanius, R. A., Terpou, B. A., & McKinnon, M. C. (2020). The sense of self in the aftermath of trauma: lessons from the default mode network in posttraumatic stress disorder. *European journal of psychotraumatology*, 11(1), 1807703. https://doi.org/10.1080/20008198.2020.1807703

3. Ideno, Y., Hayashi, K., Abe, Y., Ueda, K., Iso, H., Noda, M., Lee, J. S., & Suzuki, S. (2017). Blood pressure-lowering effect of Shinrin-yoku (Forest bathing): a systematic review and meta-analysis. *BMC complementary and alternative medicine*, 17(1), 409. https://doi.org/10.1186/s12906-017-1912-z

Chapter 16
Sound Therapies

Healing through listening and absorbing certain frequencies has become a popular choice for complementary wellness. It is relatively safe and easy to use. While most sound therapy is well tolerated, some things can be taken into consideration in order to provide the best experience possible.

There is evidence that sound may directly affect the nervous system and its ability to reset after trauma. Harnessing the parts of sound that can help to more carefully tune the vagus nerve and other parts of the body is a powerful concept. Trauma-informed herbalists may not always use sound therapy, but I encourage you to explore vibrations and music as an option for your clients.

Music is an integral part of my family's existence. I'm the least talented musician in my family, but I play the flute as well as Lizzo (or Ian Anderson, for my classic rock friends). My dad is a master guitarist, luthier, and songwriter. My closest cousin has a Master's in Piano Performance and that's the *least* of her music related accomplishments. Although it isn't a conscious thought in many of my family members' minds, I come from a family that embraces sound for its healing properties.

But you do not have to have fancy degrees or years of experience to get healing and enjoyment from sound. If you are not already incorporating some version of sound therapy into your own healing journey, I encourage you to reconsider. Surrounding yourself with music and healing vibrations is a simple way to support your body, mind, and soul.

As you read through this chapter, think about how you can get creative with this work. There are very few situations in which sound healing is contraindicated. There are many ways you can play with these ideas to create offerings and healing practices that can make a difference for you and your clients.

Thoughts on sound baths

Sound baths are amazing healing options that can allow people to relax and embrace the resetting of their nervous system. You can use all kinds of tools such as gongs, singing bowls, and recordings to create unique healing opportunities. If you haven't experienced a sound bath, find someone near you who offers them and go try a few sessions.

Many of the same recommendations I made about meditation in chapter thirteen can be applied to sound bath sessions. Offering options such as allowing people to keep their eyes open with a softened gaze may be helpful. Not cutting the lights completely off is always a best practice.

Make it clear that students can sit up whenever they need. I have students that like to sit up throughout the entire sound bath. Others have found it helpful to sit up when they feel activated, lying back down as it feels right. Verbal permission at the beginning of class helps students to feel empowered to make decisions that feel best for their body.

If you have a group setting, you may want to ask everyone to stay on their mat until the end of the session. Similar to yoga nidra, people are in a vulnerable and open state during sound baths. Encouraging people to move about as little as possible can help everyone remain in a calm space.

Singing bowls

Singing bowls are popular options for sound baths and chakra healing sessions. Traditional singing bowls are made of different types of metal and are hand hammered. Other singing bowls are made out of glass or crystal. Whatever medium your bowl is made from, the resonance that can envelope the entire room makes them a powerful ally in healing.

Lots of theories abound as to why singing bowls can be such an effective therapy for some people. There are ideas around the bowls mimicking different brain waves, so perhaps they help bring our brains into those meditative wave patterns. Maybe it is more ethereal, with the bowls addressing the etheric layers of our life force energy. Whatever the mechanism, singing bowls are one of my favorite sound healing instruments.

Many people use singing bowls to mark the beginning and end of meditation practice. During my yoga classes, I sometimes like to play them for a few minutes during savasana . I also like to employ singing bowls at the beginning and end of my energy healing sessions.

Whatever I do, I let clients know ahead of time about the plan. Remember: surprises are rarely welcome. Singing bowls have such a strong resonance that it can be jolting if it is unexpected. We want people to have a powerful experience: not a retraumatizing one!

I also use singing bowls to charge my dried herbs and herbal extracts. Tinctures, glycerites, oils, and flower essences all seem to benefit from sound baths. I try to choose an intention that matches the client's emotional needs. For instance, if they are having trouble trusting their decisions, I may choose to charge the herbs with a singing bowl attuned to the third eye for its intuitive properties.

My singing bowls are loosely tuned to the C scale. At the end of this chapter, I will discuss the C scale in relation to the chakras. There are many different frequencies that can be helpful, and some people will swear by the different frequencies for certain therapeutic benefits. What I have found to be more important than using certain frequencies is to intuitively use what you are drawn to. This seems to be true for many of the sound healing options available.

Tuning forks

Tuning forks are another vibrational healing option that I frequently employ. Eileen McKusik's book, Tuning the Human Biofield, digs deep into the practice of using tuning forks for healing. Tuning forks are easy to take along with you and they are relatively inexpensive to acquire.

As with singing bowls, there are a variety of frequencies available. There are a lot of theories regarding each frequency and how it could be employed. Play with this and see what feels right for you and your clients. I keep notes on who likes what - different people and different environments might lead me to use different forks. Emotional preferences can change your recommendations, but other issues can crop up as well.

Sometimes it's a matter of practical preference. My husband and I found that we dislike the heart chakra fork in our house. It is the exact same frequency as the hum of our air conditioner. Any time we use that particular tuning fork, we struggle to stop noticing the AC noise afterward. It's maddening. So I don't use the heart chakra tuning fork at home.

Whatever you choose for frequencies, know that the resonance will help to remove blocks and encourage better energy flow. The aura can be cleared, chakras can be realigned, and even acupressure points can be activated. All of these techniques are extremely easy to implement and many people report results after the first session. Try different techniques and find which ones resonate most with you.

Aura clearing can be easily achieved by striking the tuning fork so it hums, then sweeping through the air around a person. If you notice the sound of the tuning fork becoming muffled or distorted, hold the fork in that area longer. Once the sound becomes clear, you can begin sweeping once more.

Chakra balancing can come from specific resonances, but it can also come from pointing the tuning fork in the direction of the chakra that needs support. Rotating the fork in a clockwise motion may help add energy and a counterclockwise motion may release excess energy. I also like to move the fork up and down the midline, encouraging the connection between the chakras to be restored.

As I am a Capricorn and enjoy complicated techniques, I love addressing acupressure points with tuning forks. There are many books available that discuss different ways to employ acupressure for emotional healing techniques. Activating the tuning fork and then gently holding it on an acupressure point until it stops vibrating is a powerful healing option. No needles and a much faster result than acupuncture? I love it.

Drumming circles

Drumming circles could be an amazing offering for clients. There are a lot of people who report feeling more connected and aware of others' needs after consistently attending drumming circles. Just the co-regulation that comes from being in sync with others' movement is reason enough to consider drumming as a trauma-informed practitioner.

Drums and other percussion type instruments are relatively inexpensive and easy to access for many people. Drum circles can be a great way for deaf or hearing impaired people to participate in sound healing. The rhythms can be seen and felt, and the experience is easily adjusted for each person's needs.

Circles can be as loosely planned as everyone getting together and just drumming random beats. This alone can be enough to create that sense of connection and foster creativity. Many people will find this type of drum circle works well for them.

You can also create themed circles. These are sessions where you get together and set a theme or intention. Then each person gets a chance to drum a rhythm they associate with an emotion connected to that theme. For instance, the theme might be the heart chakra and I might choose to drum a beat I connect with unconditional love. The next person may choose the feeling of compassion and then they will drum a beat that they connect with that sensation.

Get creative. Maybe you have some Reiki friends who would like to explore merging Reiki healing circles with a drum circle. Perhaps it is a tea party slash drum circle event with herbs that match your theme. There are so many ways that this could become interactive and bring in other healing practices.

The more frequently the drumming circles get together, the more beneficial the results may be. You may find that encouraging a group to meet monthly could be a feasible option for many people. These meetings can become places where connections create healing and a sense of safety for many.

Even if you're in an area where only a few people are available to do drumming, this support option may be helpful. Although I tend to think of drumming circles as being upwards of ten to fifteen people, that doesn't mean you have to go big or go home. There are people beginning to study one on one drumming sessions with positive results.

Smaller groups may also help

Dr. Jessica Hoggle, LICSW, took inspiration from research into polyvagal theory and drumming circles and applied it to individual client interaction[1]. She found that her participants came away with a sense of how to better face discomfort. They also reported feeling that they were moving toward growth and connection.

Please note, this was a therapeutic environment and Dr. Hoggle was specifically working with clients who had been processing their trauma in a therapy setting for a while. Therefore, I'm not suggesting that we should go out and start drumming one on one to process trauma. However, we can recognize that even smaller settings can allow for similar benefits to the larger drumming circles.

There is significant evidence that drumming and using percussive instruments to create rhythmic expressions of emotions can be helpful. Whether you're creating large events with lots of people or small groups of interconnectivity, drumming can be a beneficial tool. This is an accessible, helpful option for people that are struggling with unresolved trauma.

Singing is beneficial too

As I mentioned in chapter 14, mantras are an amazing option to support a relaxed state. Long tones appear to help regulate the vagus nerve when someone is struggling with unresolved trauma. Humming and singing can also help to soothe the nervous system. Singing in a group can combine this regulation with connection.

We seem to naturally be drawn to the voice to bring a sense of peace. Singing and chanting can be found throughout many religious and spiritual groups. Because the vagus nerve is so interconnected with the signals that are sent to our larynx and pharynx, it is little surprise that singing is so helpful.

This isn't just a physical reaction. The throat chakra is also activated when we sing. Trauma itself can cause a person to stop embracing their voice. Even once the trauma is over, there is a ripple effect that can make it hard for someone to reclaim their communication.

Unresolved trauma can be an uncomfortable thing to witness. If you witness others' reactions to your unresolved trauma, it can cause you to feel as if you are not being heard or acknowledged. Reclaiming the power of the throat chakra can help a person embrace a sensation that their voice has meaning.

Singing doesn't have to be beautiful to be beneficial. The advent of social media has created a performative environment that can lead us to subconsciously believe something is worthless if it isn't perfect. This is far from true. We can sing to our plants, hum to our animals, or just belt a tune out at any time for the fun of it.

When I recommend singing to clients, they can sometimes be taken aback by the suggestion. However, many people have songs they love. They may be willing to sing lullabies to their favorite plant. Again, we're back to the theme of this chapter: get creative and find things that work for you and your clients!

Frequencies for the chakras

In the last chapter, we discussed a bit about chakra balancing and its usefulness for trauma support. In chapter ten, we saw which essential oil scent families could be helpful for their corresponding chakras. One final aspect of chakra balancing is utilizing different sounds for chakra support.

There are different frequencies that have been associated with the chakras. I have a tuning fork set that has some of these more complex frequencies. However, I have found the most benefit in focusing on the basic C-scale association.

The C-scale association assigns one note of the C scale to each of the chakras. The root is C, sacral is D, solar plexus E, heart F, throat G, third eye A, and crown B. Single tones can be helpful, but I have enjoyed playing with the corresponding key signatures to create specific balancing effects.

For instance, G major helps to build energy up in the throat chakra. G minor helps the throat chakra to release excess energy. Similarly to an alterative herb that restores balance, neither scale pushes the chakra out of alignment. The G minor scale may help release excess energy, but it doesn't continue to sap energy out of the throat chakra once it is in balance.

This means the vibrational patterns of different songs can be helpful without being damaging. I've played with different chord progressions to create music that can support balancing in multiple chakra centers. For you other music nerds, I encourage you to experiment with this. See if there is a chord progression that you like that could be used to create a meditation song specifically to balance the chakras with which you are struggling.

Making meditation music

Furthermore, fellow music lovers, I encourage you to look into making your own songs. As a hobby, I create meditation music. Some of the songs are not that great and others make it into my playlist for classes.

Making your own music is useful on several fronts. First of all, I am inspired by my students and I love tailoring songs that match the guided meditations I craft for them. Secondly, I can use the music without paying for usage rights. Third, it's a great time to tap into creativity and give yourself a dopamine boost from playing around with your instruments.

When composing meditation music, I look for simple, repeatable themes. I also tend to use longer tones and less melodies. Depending on the reason I am creating the music, I may add in nature sounds. My backyard birds are grateful for the fancier feed I get after I've made a commission using their song.

Humans perceive many high- and low- frequencies as indications of danger. I find myself drawn to using my alto flute and my viola more than my regular flute and violin during meditation music sessions. It seems that the higher frequencies of the latter can bring a person back to a state of alertness and the lower frequencies of the former keep a person more securely focused in their meditative state.

Play with this. There are different synthesizer sounds and interesting ways to record. I bring in the singing bowls and tuning forks when I have the chance. There is no wrong way to approach making music, there just may be ways that are best for you and your clients.

Choosing music for class

We talked in chapter six about choosing instrumental music for the waiting area. In trauma-informed settings, I almost always default to instrumental pieces. However, I know many people love to use more popular types of music for classes. You may choose songs with lyrics or well known tunes that can evoke memories and emotions.

When you do this, consider the lyrics of the songs you have chosen. Do they possibly contain thoughts or phrases that could trigger traumatic memories? What is the general message of the music you have chosen?

As I have mentioned several times, it is impossible to plan for everyone's response. However, a bit of careful planning can help us create an environment that allows people to better focus on their healing. Music and sound have the capability of creating a healing effect on the nervous system - let's commit to making sure everyone can lean into that effect as much as possible.

Choosing music for you

When looking at music for yourself, think about what you regularly consume. I believe that the main quality of our music should be that it enriches our lives. Is it uplifting? Toxic?

Music can help us explore deep, sometimes sombering, topics. It can also be uplifting and joyful. If I consciously choose music for my edification, I feel better. Think carefully about the lyrics of songs you are listening to and consider how your music is contributing to your healing.

I'm not suggesting we should all listen to upbeat pop every day. Do not misconstrue my words as a vote for toxic positivity. However, if we choose to constantly consume music with themes of violence and hate, our minds may struggle to recover. Just pay attention to what you're allowing yourself to absorb. We can do similar things with our TV shows and social media feed. Mindful consumption can be healing!

Reference

1. Hoggle, 2022 POLYVAGAL-INFORMED THERAPEUTIC DRUMMING FOR VICTIMS OF INTERPERSONAL VIOLENCE: A FEASIBILITY STUDY

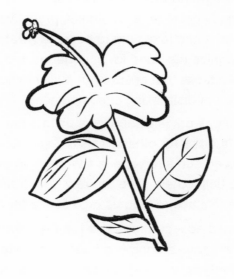

Chapter 17
Self Evaluation
and Care

Our work as trauma-informed herbalists means that we must be in the right headspace to hold space for others. We must consistently practice mindfulness, proactively plan for our emotional needs, and take time to become aware of our biases. We must recognize the need for boundaries and implement consistent care tasks that ensure our ability to support others who are victims of distressing circumstances.

Our inner work is what allows us to create effective healing opportunities for others. This doesn't mean we have to have it all figured out: everyone is a work in progress. However, it is difficult to help others if we are raw from trauma and do not have systems in place to help us hold space for others.

When we accept a role as a trauma-informed practitioner, we make a choice to bear witness to all kinds of suffering. Actively scheduling self care helps to reduce stress and burnout. In order to continue holding space for others and taking care of our own health, we must consider ways to reduce secondary trauma in ourselves.

Do your inner work

Doing inner work to recognize bias, reduce your trauma response, and become a neutral source for others is a vital part of offering trauma-informed care. This inner work is a necessary part of your commitment to your health and your clients' well being. You cannot be an effective practitioner if you avoid taking stock of your own beliefs, judgments, and mental well being.

Trauma-informed herbalists have the added responsibility to be working on their own healing. Clearing mental blocks, recognizing internalized bias, and working to practice what we preach are important aspects of self care. I encourage you to read through this section and find at least two things to implement as you work toward being better prepared to offer support to clients.

These practices can help anyone to grow a stronger sense of empathy and well being. Even if you're not looking to take on clients anytime soon, think about these ideas and see what could be helpful for you. The world is always a better place when we choose empathy toward each other.

Internalized bias

Self evaluation helps everyone, but these practices can be extremely beneficial to those of us with some form of privilege. It can help us to notice internalized bias, slow down our reactions, and choose a response that is healing instead of damaging. This is a lifelong study and everyone can benefit from recognizing their biases.

Reactions that come from subconscious bias can occur when we encounter a situation that is contrary to our lived experience. Many times people who hold some form of privilege may be blind to others' experiences. If you are white, male, straight, or cis-gendered, it may be difficult to see the struggles of a person who is BIPOC, female, or LGBTQ+.

Are you unconvinced that you suffer from internalized bias? Dianne Bondy, a black yoga teacher and accessibility educator introduced me to Harvard's implicit association tests. I encourage you to check them out. They have gender, race, skin tone, and fat bias tests. It might surprise you to find that you don't pass them as well as you expect. It was eye opening when halfway through the first test I tried, I could tell I was failing due to my slowing reaction times.

Don't be upset if you fail these internalized bias tests. Instead, use that knowledge to recognize when you might be inclined to make a snap judgment about someone because of these biases. Remember these failures when someone tells you about a situation and your knee-jerk reaction is disbelief.

These tests can help you recognize that your disbelief may be coming from a place of subconscious bias. When you notice this, it becomes easier to momentarily release the disbelief and offer a neutral place of support that will support your client.

The effect of secondary trauma

Secondary trauma occurs in many people who support victims of trauma. Hearing about traumatic experiences and witnessing the aftermath of trauma is a difficult thing. As a trauma-informed practitioner, you may hear about terrifying situations. You may bear witness to something that activates your trauma memories. These feelings can create a situation in which you begin to experience symptoms of trauma.

The sooner you recognize that secondary trauma could affect you, the better prepared you can be to get support. Knowing this effect is real and proactively finding ways to mitigate your body's stress and responses can make a big difference. The first thing that you can do is become aware of the somatic responses your body has when you become stressed.

Once you're aware of the responses that tell you when you may be approaching dysregulation, thinking about your alertness on a scale of one to ten may help you notice when you need more breaks to come back into your window of tolerance. On this scale, one is a state of hypoarousal. The freeze response has kicked in completely and the dorsal vagal state is most active. Around four, five, and six are the ventral vagal moments of safety and connectedness. Ten is a complete state of hyperarousal. The sympathetic system is in control.

Taking time throughout the day and noting where you are on this scale can help you catch things before they cause you to spiral. There may be moments where you are able to choose a break because you've noticed your body moving one direction or the other on the arousal scale. Having techniques to help you ground and center can help keep you in balance.

When you notice that you are in a state of dysregulation, what do you do to bring yourself back? Can you name five different techniques that could help you recenter and come back into your window of tolerance? Perhaps there is an essential oil that you are attracted to for support. Maybe certain breathing techniques are comforting for you. Come up with a list of soothing practices and the next time you notice yourself feeling dysregulated, try them out and see how they help.

Self regulation is a great starting point, but it only goes so far. Enlisting the help of professionals to care for you as you are supporting others is extremely important. I encourage all of my wellness practitioner students to go ahead and start working with a therapist. Even if you don't feel you *need* someone right now, go ahead and find someone that you can start seeing so you have that support.

Start therapy NOW - don't wait until you're in emergency mode

One of the best decisions I have ever made was to get myself a therapist *before* I found myself in a situation that activated my trauma. I was able to take some time and find someone whose therapy style worked best for me. My therapist also understood my baseline feelings and reactions to situations. This meant that when I ended up in a situation that activated my anxiety, she was able to see the differences firsthand. This made our sessions more effective.

If you proactively look for a therapist, you're more likely to find someone that fits your needs. Find yourself a therapist that resonates with you. If you have to "therapist shop", that's fine. Sometimes it takes meeting two or three people before you find someone that feels right. Don't be afraid to state how you feel sessions would benefit you the most. Let them know if you prefer homework or are just coming in to decompress.

Certain forms of therapy may be more effective than others for you. At different points in my healing, cognitive behavioral therapy (CBT) has been helpful. At other times, I find a more bottom up approach such as EMDR is more useful. I'm lucky in that my therapist is also well versed in polyvagal theory and she helps me find related exercises that fit my needs.

Therapy is a safe space for you to work through feelings and concerns. This is where you can discuss the reactions you had to someone sharing their experiences. You can talk about the problems you're facing and the traumas you've experienced because this is your time. A good therapist will create space for your needs during your sessions.

Your therapist can also help you come up with other tools to be more mindful of somatic sensations and emotions that may arise. They can help you to find new ways to address hypo- or hyper- arousal as it occurs. They can be a sounding board for when you're unsure of how to proceed with your own mental health care. Most therapists will introduce you to complementary tools that can enhance your therapy

Journaling and self help apps

Your therapist may encourage you to keep a journal of how you feel in between your sessions. Journaling can be a great way for us to sort through thoughts and express ourselves. It can also be a useful tool to take to therapy to discuss recurring patterns you notice in your thought process.

Some apps may be useful in getting us to take a break and be mindful of our emotions throughout the day. There are many different apps available that can complement the work you do with your therapist. I have found I enjoy the CBT Thought Diary app. The free version has a useful guide to help you think through your emotions and thought processes. The paid version has a lot of interesting bells and whistles, but isn't necessary.

I stay busy and struggle to slow down sometimes. Having a journal available to write in or receiving the notifications from the Thought Diary app helps me to check in and see how I'm doing. I encourage you to find something similar to help remind you to check in with yourself.

Complementary therapies work for you too

Finding other practitioners who work in complementary fields can help you to enhance your healing experience. You may choose a different practitioner or modality depending on what you are experiencing on an ongoing basis. Taking time to address self care through complementary modalities helps to strengthen a mind-body-spirit balance that can help you feel safe and secure.

Massage therapists, yoga teachers, other herbalists, Reiki masters, and acupuncturists may be some of the options available to you. Find someone you trust and that you believe will keep your information private. Feeling safe and connected with professional practitioners can help you to relax and enjoy the healing process more.

Massage therapy can help to release physical tension that is caused by stressful days. This is an oversimplification of the benefits of this modality, but it best describes why I find it helpful. I encourage you to consider some form of massage as part of your healing regimen.

A massage therapist may be able to help you pinpoint where you hold tension in your body. They may also give you ideas as to how you can reduce that tension in between sessions. The extensive understanding massage therapists have of the musculoskeletal system makes them an amazing resource for tension related aches and pains.

Finding a yoga or tai chi class that you can take routinely will promote connectedness and mind-body healing. Taking a class allows you to melt into the background and focus on yourself. Accepting the support and healing that occurs can go a long way toward building resilience.

Many of the yoga and tai chi classes I've attended help to activate the ventral vagal response. Different poses, synchronized movements, and breathwork can help to bring that feeling of safety and connection to your mat. Even on weeks when I don't feel I have time to take a class, I always feel better if I go ahead and commit to my practice.

Herbalists are another fantastic option. Working with another herbalist may feel odd at first, but I highly recommend it. Having an outside perspective on your wellbeing can help to offer you support systems you never would have considered for yourself. I love having a consult and getting an epiphany as we work through my current symptom set.

You don't have to see someone on a frequent basis for this to be beneficial. If you have someone in your area that you trust, I encourage you to set up quarterly appointments. Just having someone to brainstorm with who speaks your "lingo" can be very helpful.

My Reiki practitioner is a vital part of my healing. Find someone who can work on your energy, such as a chakra healer or acupuncturist. Having someone who supports you on that subtle energy layer can bring healing you would not have otherwise found.

Vital life force energy, qi, or prana, is sometimes overlooked as we make our way through the physical world. I encourage you to work with some energy healing specialists and see what you experience. It can bring breakthroughs and inspiration in ways that other modalities cannot.

Whatever you choose, make a commitment to consistently work with someone. Even if it takes a couple of trials to find a person you trust and connect with, give yourself the gift of that conscious effort. You will thank me when you're becoming a stronger, more powerful healer while also taking care of yourself!

Holding space as a neutral observer

A final aspect of self evaluation that I want to address is your ability to hold space as a neutral observer. I saved this for last because it is difficult to hold this space if you're not working to be aware of your bias, seeing a therapist consistently, and finding help through other practitioners. Holding space is an important aspect of being a trauma-informed herbalist, as our judgments and personal beliefs can stop a person from receiving the healing they deserve.

When I hold space, I am not trying to force myself to not feel anything. Instead, I am working to notice feelings that may come up in order to not react to those feelings. I work to filter my responses and questions through empathy and neutrality so that my judgments and opinions are less likely to affect my work.

Ego has no place in our consultations. If you find yourself wanting to press a point to prove you're the best practitioner, your ego is clouding your ability to hold space. If you worry about saying something because you are afraid of looking silly, you're allowing your ego to interfere. Focus on your client and their needs during your sessions.

This is a lifelong study that can be applied in so many aspects of our journey. The longer I practice, the better I find myself able to hold space for people with differing opinions or who come from situations that are vastly different from my lived experience. I am less likely to encroach on a conversation with a list of items I think a person should do. Instead, I find myself a better listener and stronger observer than ever.

Self care

Self evaluation is important. Sometimes heavy work must be done in order to advance and become a better person. However, balance must be struck. Self care is the other side of this coin. It isn't always about pushing to restructure ourselves. There are also periods of rest and relaxation that allow us to integrate the new lessons we have learned.

Some of the complementary practitioners I named earlier in this chapter are part of your self care. Accepting healing and care without feeling the need to *do* anything to be worthy of this care can go a long way. We can also implement plant healing ideas found earlier in this book. We may also find benefit in nurturing connection with others, and participating in retreats designed for us to accept healing and love.

As you've read through this text, I have no doubt you've come across some herbs, essential oils, and flower essences that you thought, "oh, that's for me!" I encourage you to implement these things! You are worthy of healing and rest. You deserve to give yourself the same kind of care you are giving to your clients.

The mindful tea exercise I outline in chapter thirteen is my favorite self care ritual. I start all of my herbal students on this exercise rather quickly when they work with me. I believe it allows us a chance to connect deeply with the herbs while also checking in with ourselves.

Consciously planning to connect with others who help us feel safe and loved is important. I have certain friends that activate my ventral vagal system for certain aspects of my life. I encourage you to think about who supports that feeling of community for you and nurture those friendships.

Also be conscious of the media you consume. You may spend a lot of time online, lamenting the curated feeds on Instagram and Tiktok. I have a horrible habit of bingeing true crime documentaries. Pay attention to what you are focusing on and shift it when necessary so that you can more easily return to that state of ventral vagal safety.

Attending workshops and healing retreats where you can focus on your own healing is one of my favorite things. I challenge you to find a retreat that is only for you. Don't think about how you can take the information home and implement it into your business. Just go for yourself. The freedom of just focusing inward for a bit is refreshing.

There are so many ways we can focus on self improvement, evaluation, and care. These aspects are necessary in order to help us stay grounded and feeling safe, even as we witness horrendous accounts of trauma and pain. If we are deliberate in our plans, we can find a rewarding, healing career in trauma-informed herbalism.

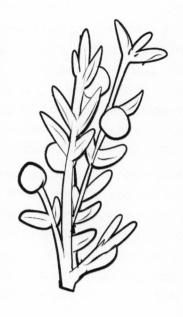

Chapter 18
Connecting to the Wellness Community

One of the daunting tasks of being a trauma-informed herbalist can be trying to find other practitioners and therapists that will become part of your referral network. It may feel overwhelming to try to determine which doctors are herb-friendly and which ones will yell at your clients for considering supplements. You may even struggle with imposter syndrome, not knowing what would be the best way to present your information to someone in an allopathic, clinical setting.

Building relationships with other professionals and having collaborations that support their clients as well as yours is extremely beneficial for everyone when done correctly. I encourage you to start a list of local (and virtual) practitioners that have specializations that complement your work. Start reaching out and building relationships in order to strengthen your connection and discover how your clients could benefit from their offerings.

Building relationships with other professionals

It's important to not create these lists of helpful practitioners with a "set it and forget it" mindset. Working to build relationships with other professionals is important. Reach out and invite people to relationship building sessions. These sessions can be as simple as meeting some of your fellow healers for tea or coffee. They can be as complex as a monthly meetup of wellness practitioners with different themes and speakers.

These relationships can be as beneficial for us as they are for our clients. As a 911 dispatcher, I quickly learned that no one else in the world "gets it" as well as other dispatchers. I had friendships with dispatchers that I wouldn't trade for anything. No one else understands the nuances of being at a console, trying to determine how to best help the person on the other end of the phone or radio.

Natural health practices are similar. You will find that other herbalists, yoga instructors, and natural wellness community leaders are able to better sympathize with the weird quirks of our industry. No one else understands the obstacles we face as well as others in the field.

Conventional medicine doctors may be more difficult to connect with, as they stay very busy. However, I have had a good response from a few that are interested in integrative or functional medicine. I don't necessarily have long conversations and brainstorming sessions with these doctors, but I do find it helpful to know which ones run the herb-friendly practices in my area.

You will also find that some of these relationships will naturally segue into partnerships that create amazing collaborative opportunities. Some of the best brainstorms I have are when I'm sitting around talking with other yoga instructors or herbalists. See these relationships as a way to better serve your community as a whole through strong partnerships.

Workshops and other collaborations

Workshops and other collaborations such as podcast interviews can be an amazing way to get your message out. This can be a strong way to build your relationship with other professionals while also giving your clients an extra taste of your work. Brainstorm with some of your closer colleagues and see if there are interesting ways that your work could intersect!

Make sure your collaborations are to the benefit of your clients. Don't partner with anyone and everyone. I'm guilty of getting excited when I make goals to work with __ number of people in a quarter and not being careful to curate the list to my clients' needs. What I find is that the collaborations that do not benefit my clients tend to fall flat and not gain traction.

I love collaborations because I know I have fans that love me but will never take that step to work with me. However, there are other professionals who just happen to have the right message for those fans. If I can collaborate with the other professionals, these fans will take the next step with those professionals and make the commitment to heal.

The inverse is also true: these other professionals have fans who will recognize me as the next step on their healing journey and they begin to work with me. This means that more people are being helped by the right practitioners. More people are finding ways to heal and bring themselves into a safer place so that trauma responses (and other concerns) can be resolved!

When collaborations go sour

Sometimes collaborations don't work out. I will never forget when I reached out to a local practitioner to collaborate on a project. We had discussed it over coffee in the past and it seemed like the perfect time to move forward with the workshop series.

I mentioned the venue that was happy to host the two of us and she told me she would think about it. The next thing I know, she's gone behind my back and booked the venue by herself. She never reached out to explain, never apologized, just took the space from me and never looked back.

This backfired on her, as I will never again work with her. She also ended up not having much participation in the classes she booked and I haven't heard much about her since. This incident hurt me but there was no lasting damage in my world.

I pray that she finds a way to overcome her hangups and is able to start helping people again. Her proposed niche was amazing and I'm disappointed in how this turned out. Thanks to her actions toward me, I'm now unable to recommend her to certain clients that could benefit from the work she purported to offer.

I can only speculate on why this person pulled such a stunt, but I have seen my students hesitate to work with others. Usually hesitation comes from a place of imposter syndrome. There may be a worry around not being able to keep up with the other presenter. Or worry that power dynamics could affect the outcome. There also are some people who are worried that they will lose clients to the other presenter.

Everyone is having similar worries and things sometimes do go wrong. But at the end of the day, if you continue to work hard and form healthy collaborative partnerships, things tend to work themselves out. Continue forming these partnerships out of love of your clients and enjoyment of sharing the work you do and watch the healing you facilitate resonate out into the world and down through the generations.

Be willing to refer out

Recognize that a deeper mind-body-spirit healing can occur when a person has access to multiple high quality practitioners and resources. Do not hesitate to give your clients access to other practitioners that can help them on their journey. You are not expected to do it all and no one *can* do it all.

In my world, I rarely use the phrase "referring out" to mean dismissing a person and sending them elsewhere. Occasionally that happens, but more often I find myself recommending a client go work with a yoga therapist for a few weeks before returning to regroup with me. I have become as much of a reference section for outside resources as a healer myself.

Referral sheets

Instead of trying to look up every single person's contact info, I like to have referral sheets on hand. I have a couple of different types of referral sheets, but I encourage you to start with just one and expand as needed. This referral sheet is usually one page, focused on available herb-friendly physicians, therapists, complementary healers, public health resources, and support groups in the area.

Start your referral sheet by sitting down and thinking about who you know. Are there practitioners that you have met that would be helpful to have on your referral sheet? Are there people who you have built relationships with that have beneficial services to your community? Be picky: my referral lists only have practitioners that I feel confident will have my clients' best interests at heart.

Next, you will make a list of people that you've heard people speak of in a positive manner. Perhaps a friend mentioned a massage therapist that has a welcoming practice. Maybe another practitioner was singing the praises of a physician. These people can start to fill in the gaps for types of practitioners you may not know personally but would be beneficial for your clients.

Finally, make a list of people who seem to have a good reputation. Try to connect with these practitioners to get a feel for their work. If you can't get in contact with them, check around with friends or look for online reviews to see if there are any red flags. If not, you can use this group of people to help fill out the remaining gaps on your referral sheet.

Once you have your referral sheet in a draft form, take some time to consider race and gender biases that are appearing on your list. Look at how you could diversify and amplify voices of phenomenal practitioners you did not consider at first glance. Many of your clients can benefit from diversity in their healing team, but may not know that these practitioners exist.

Once your referral sheet is complete, start using it! Look over this list every six months and update it where necessary. Maybe you've met someone at a local event that could be a better fit than the current practitioner on your list. Perhaps one of the functional medicine doctors is so full they are no longer taking clients. Someone else may be taking time off from their practice. Work to keep this list up to date so it stays helpful for your clients.

Specialized referral sheets

I encourage you to start with the generalized referral sheet and add to your collection as it seems appropriate. As I mentioned earlier in this chapter, I have a few different specialized referral sheets. As you grow, you may find yourself drawn to working with people who have certain types of trauma or other concerns. You may find that a specialized referral sheet can be beneficial for your clients in those situations.

You could create specialized referral sheets for several situations. Think of things such as birth trauma (or postnatal care in general), specific chronic illnesses, adoption trauma, military related trauma, and intimate partner violence. It can be helpful to list therapists and healers that have specific training in helping with the concern.

Then add public health offerings, support groups, and other community offerings that could support someone dealing with that particular issue. Depending on what the specialization is, you may find online offerings that could help as well. Get creative and find several different forms of support.

Considering mental health recommendations

If you have nothing else on your recommendation sheet, I encourage you to list different therapists you can recommend.

Therapists can come in many forms, so check your local laws for what constitutes a mental health professional. Bonus points for any therapists that have a speciality that your clients need.

There are many different ways that therapists can specialize. There are different types of training that one can take in order to be able to successfully work with different concerns. For instance, someone with adoption trauma may have a different set of needs than someone who has suffered from intimate partner violence.

I encourage you to have each therapist labeled on your recommendation sheet for their specialities. This makes it easier to quickly highlight a couple of options that might be helpful for the client that is currently sitting across from you. It also makes it easier for clients to choose a therapist if they have undisclosed concerns.

Therapists make up the majority of my recommendation sheet's mental health section, but I do occasionally recommend psychiatrists when a client is looking for help with medication. Psychiatrists may be a little trickier for your area, as many are uncomfortable with herbal supplementation because of how little evidence we have on how herbs interact with psychotropics. Most therapists will have recommendations for psychiatrists for their clients, so I rarely find myself having that conversation.

Other support systems

Therapy is not the end of the healing work someone can access. Of course, therapy is the appropriate place to process through certain traumas and learn techniques that can help to resolve memories. However, we have many other support systems that can be offered to clients.

Another large section on my recommendation sheet is for support groups. There are all kinds of support groups that are available and many meet virtually as well as in person. I list the group name, a contact number, and the day/time they meet each month.

Sometimes these groups will even ask you to come speak on your work and how it relates to their situation. I encourage you to consider going, even if they ask for you to do it on a volunteer basis. You never know when you are offering encouragement to someone who might otherwise feel hopeless.

Public health services and community offerings such as food banks, church ministries, and wellness programs for under-supported communities can go on your list as well. In more rural areas, there might not be many candidates. In bigger cities, these offerings tend to feel endless, so I encourage you to find ones that you've witnessed in action or heard good reviews about them.

There are many other modalities you may want to add to this list. Yoga therapists, music therapists, and massage therapists could be beneficial. Acupuncturists, tai chi classes, and naturopathic physicians in your area could also help. Find the highest quality options and try to offer a variety of support options on your referral list.

Referrals that don't help

Occasionally I will build a relationship with a practitioner, only to find out from clients that they have done more harm than good in a session. I always take my clients' reviews into account when updating my referral sheets. If one or two people mention not enjoying sessions, I recognize that it might be a personality difference causing the dissonance.

If several clients come back saying they did not enjoy the practitioner's work, I consider that a good enough reason to remove them from my referral sheet. They may be perfectly fine healers for some, but they don't fit my clients' needs. This doesn't stand as a judgment on that person, they just may not be what my clients are needing at this time.

There are other times where someone comes back to me after an experience that was so toxic that I need to immediately remove the practitioner from my referral list. I also inform other practitioners if I have recommended the practitioner to them in the past. I tend to leave details off and just mention that a client has had a toxic interaction and that we have concerns.

As trauma-informed herbalists, we want to keep others safe, but we do not want to participate in gossip. If you run into someone who has created a toxic experience for a client, use your judgment to determine if other healers in the community need to be made aware. This is a hard topic to summarize in a single paragraph. We always want to bring abuse to light, but not all negative situations are abusive. Use mindful discernment to determine what details need to be shared and who needs the information. We are healers, not destroyers.

Final thoughts

Connecting to others in the wellness industry is an important part of maximizing your effectiveness for your clients and community. Not only can you find healing and support from others who understand the obstacles of being a natural practitioner, you can optimize your clients' experiences during the healing process.

Take the time to learn who your trustworthy, high quality local colleagues are. Only recommend practitioners that you are confident will be helpful for your clients. Don't hesitate to take someone off your recommendation list if they are not supporting your clients the way they need to.

When you find colleagues that you connect with, you will find ways to collaborate with each other and create amazing offerings for your communities. Work to create strong bonds of trust, be transparent, and support each other on this path. There is more than enough abundance to go around if we all work together.

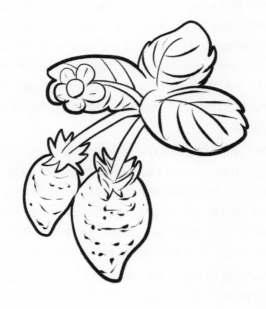

Chapter 19
Considering Marginalized Groups

I write this chapter to try to bring attention to the fact that trauma-informed practitioners must consider the needs of marginalized groups. However, I am unable to speak for many of the groups I will mention here. I encourage you to do further research into the different topics we discuss in this chapter and take the time to listen to those who have firsthand knowledge of these struggles.

Listen to what the experts in these communities are asking for and then attempt to honor their requests. Don't stop there. Recognize that individuals have personal preferences and ask your clients and students what they find helpful. Use common sense and don't ask about every little thing, but do note when it could be appropriate to get individual feedback.

As with all of our work, remain humble. You may receive criticism that makes you uncomfortable. Don't react. Sit with it and remain open to any suggestions that are offered to you. Critiques and requests for accommodations can be difficult to make and we should always honor the effort someone puts in to offering feedback. See those moments as opportunities to improve your offerings.

Whenever these opportunities present themselves, learn how to respond to requests for support with grace. Making faces, changing body language or tone of voice, or huffing because you're trying to process the request can be taken as you not wanting to help. Even if the shift in your communication is based on you trying to think of how you could make something work, someone could misread it as a defensive posture. Remember, our work is to facilitate others' healings, not to prove ourselves.

Trauma affects us in different layers

Earlier in this book, we discussed the different ways trauma could be classified based on the amount and length of the traumatic experiences. Trauma can also be grouped into different layers. I've chosen to introduce this trauma classification system in this chapter because these five layers can help you better visualize how quickly trauma could build for someone who is in a marginalized community. The five layers we will discuss here are personal, family, ancestor, race, and other collective trauma.

Personal traumas are the experiences that you directly encounter in your life. They directly occur to you and may affect how you respond to future stress. You may witness an event firsthand and experience trauma. You may also hear others' experiences and find yourself struggling with secondary trauma.

Family trauma is the layer of trauma that happens to your relatives. The trauma that happens to your parents and grandparents (and to a lesser extent cousins, aunts, and uncles) can cause them to treat you differently. For instance, if your parents lost a child before raising you, they may have been overly protective. Their traumas may or may not create trauma for you, but they can definitely change your resilience and ability to stay wired for connection.

Ancestral trauma is the layer of trauma that comes from your inherited genetics and energetics. Previous generations have experienced trauma that leads to epigenetic changes. Those changes can be handed down through the generations and affect your response to stress.

In Ayurveda, there is a concept of certain energetic patterns being passed from generation to generation. Similarly to physical DNA, the idea is that these energetics affect how we respond to certain situations. Energetic imbalances can be handed down through the generations until someone works to heal them.

Racial trauma is a significant type of trauma that is often overlooked or dismissed. Here in the United States, the black, indigenous, and people of color (BIPOC) community suffers from discrimination on personal and systemic levels. This can be overt acts of abuse or assault. It can also be as subtle as policies and procedures that make accessibility more difficult.

Even the mental health related research that is available is heavily weighted toward white individuals. This means mental health diagnoses, treatments, and expected outcomes rarely account for the unique struggles that face the BIPOC community. The nuance of an individual's experience is lost and treatments are not as effective.

Other collective traumas can occur in the communities with which you are involved. Natural disasters are one example of collective trauma. Say "Katrina" and it evokes a certain response from those who lived through the events and aftermath of New Orleans flooding. Here in Alabama, you can say "April 27th" and people immediately understand you are referring to the generational event that spawned dozens of tornadoes and killed many people across our state.

Trauma that occurs to a community that faces discrimination could also fall into this layer. Both overt and systemic discrimination can create feelings of unresolved trauma. People who are disabled, part of the LGBTQ community, or are older can face discrimination as a group.

These collective traumas can occur in almost any community and can change the way the people of that community interact. A group that witnesses multiple violent events over the course of a short time frame may become fragmented and suspicious of each other. Children growing up in an unsafe neighborhood may be affected by the ongoing danger and become wired for fear. A ventral vagal state of being connected becomes even more difficult to achieve in these circumstances.

Note how the different layers of trauma can overlap. A community trauma may have aspects that also affect your family or your personal experience. Multiple traumas can combine into a complex web of reactions. Revisit this catalog of layers frequently to help you gain empathy for the subtle ways trauma can affect clients.

Be proactive

When you chose to become a trauma-informed herbalist, you made the decision to be proactive in supporting others. Pay attention to the ways you can proactively adjust your policies and procedures to help others. When you are working as a practitioner, set your feelings aside and work to notice how you can improve.

Start by listening to people who are struggling. Listen to their words and their concerns without trying to correct them. Sometimes I see social media posts by friends who are lamenting accessibility issues. The comments section on these posts can be atrocious.

People tend to go into "fix-it" mode and either suggest another way for the friend to approach the situation or they try to indicate the friend should have a better outlook toward things. Recognize that, unless the person has explicitly asked for ideas, they are trying to express their frustration at a broken system. Listen to learn how we can do better, empathize, but don't give unsolicited advice.

Another way to learn how to improve is to read books by authors of different marginalized groups. Follow them on social media. Amplify these authors' voices. Share their content with your clients. Find ways to implement their suggestions while also helping others become more conscious of the need to change.

Offering accommodations

Accommodations are an important part of trauma-informed care. Do your best to accommodate every reasonable request with eagerness. Seamless integration of accommodations means people are able to focus on their healing instead of worrying about whether or not their requests will result in poorer service. Do everything you can to prepare and execute accomodations flawlessly.

This won't always work perfectly. The first time I tried to turn on my Zoom closed captioning, I read through the instructions three times, thought I had it right, and it still didn't work. I was so embarrassed because I had a fan specifically request the accommodation and I totally botched the execution.

I was able to send the fan the transcript of the event and figured out the mistakes, but it doesn't stop the fact that now I'm another disappointment for that person. Another difficulty and frustration. I do my best to offer a seamless experience for anyone that requests help, but sometimes I mess up. When I botch something I always try to apologize, do what I can to fix it, and work towards doing better the next time.

Speak to clients who may need personalized accommodations. Speak to members of communities you serve to see if there are general accommodations you could easily put into place. Do your background research, but also reach out to hear the voices of those who are working with you.

My friend Layla is deaf. When I designed a restorative yoga class for the deaf and hard of hearing community, I reached out to her for ideas. I told her my plan and asked what she thought I could change that would help. She gave me some thoughts around how to approach the class. She mentioned how difficult it is to do yoga mindfully when you do not know how long to hold a pose, because then you're looking back over your shoulder to watch for cues that it's time to move into the next pose.

I am extremely grateful that I have friends like Layla that are able to help. However, don't rely solely on clients and friends to guide you. It is not their responsibility to educate you on their struggles. They are not here to convince you that they have experienced discrimination. When appropriate, ask what we can do to make things more accessible. Never ask why they need to be more accessible.

Recommended Reading

I initially prepared a section here discussing the different ways that race, gender, sexual orientation, or disability could cause someone to struggle. Even though I fall into certain categories, I cannot speak for everyone. Therefore I've changed my mind on how to approach this. Instead of talking more about what I know, I want to spend the remainder of this chapter listing out several books that you may find helpful. I have read many of them and have had friends recommend the rest.

"The Wake Up" by Michelle MiJung Kim

Michelle helps us to better own the act of allyship in a compassionate, humanity-focused light. The book is a heavier read, but the way she approaches the discussion around creating effective change is inspiring. Michelle has created a mindful exploration on how we can do better and I encourage you to listen.

"Diversity in Clinical Practice" by Lambers Fisher

This book addresses concerns around diversity and offers real world translations to the issues that face healing professionals in practice. He has exercises that help you to dive into a stronger self awareness around cultural competency without shaming you for the areas you need to improve. It's written from a therapist's viewpoint, but many of the issues and concerns he addresses apply to natural healers as well.

"Yoga Revolution" by Jivana Heyman

A book designed to introduce you to inclusivity as a yoga practitioner. Jivana does a fantastic job discussing ways to create an environment of service as part of your yoga practice. Although this book is aimed for the yoga crew, there are many great ideas that can be applied in an herbalist's practice. Read this book for the paradigm shift, it's worth it.

"Damaged Like Me" by Kimberly Dark

A book of essays that highlight the different ways that people in vulnerable communities find ways to heal and support each other. Resilience at its finest. Her highlights on types of discrimination that are rarely discussed, such as fat bias, are powerful.

"Decolonizing Trauma Work" by Renee Linklater

An eye opening account of how indigenous practices for wellness can be used to support trauma healing. With a focus on healing from trauma that has been imposed by colonialism, Renee addresses the need to reconnect with ancestral and cultural identity. She encourages a return to community based healing in order to reduce the need for conventional interventions.

"Whipping Girl" by Julia Serano

One of my friend Catherine's recommendations, this book explores sexism through the eyes of a transsexual woman. It drives home how pervasive misogyny is, especially in the

United States. Julia researched genetics and developmental biology for seventeen years and holds a PhD in biochemistry and molecular biophysics. The combination of her expertise and personal experience makes this a must read for anyone wanting to better understand struggles of people who are transgender.

"Seven Sisters for Seven Days" by Michelle Peterson

Not directly related to trauma, but this book offers a model for community-based postpartum care. Mindful postpartum care can help to reduce long term traumatic effects of a tough birth. Community support, when done correctly and with love, can help a person stay in a ventral vagal state during the trying "fourth trimester."

"Deaf in America" by Carol Padden and Tom Humphries

An older book, but a good introduction into understanding deaf culture. It touches on how signed languages are vital and how the hearing world's misperceptions cause so much damage. If you want to shift your perspective away from believing that hearing is a requirement for a rich life, start with this book.

"The End of Bias" by Jessica Nordell

A book that focuses on solutions to unconscious bias concerns, Jessica takes a look at several scenarios in which people have worked to overcome disparities in healthcare, law enforcement, and many other scenarios. Instead of just pointing out the problems, this book helps us to see what others are doing to stop their biases from affecting others.

Final thoughts

Trauma-informed herbalism is all about adjusting and supporting others. When a person is at risk of experiencing discrimination, it becomes twice as important that we consider their needs and be flexible. Our consideration is not going to cure everything, but it can keep from adding to the strain our clients may be already experiencing.

The pledge we take to do no harm also includes a proactive component to do better. If the book recommendations I have made here are not resonating, do some research to find other educational materials that could help. Ask friends, look to professionals, and find ways to learn how to be better.

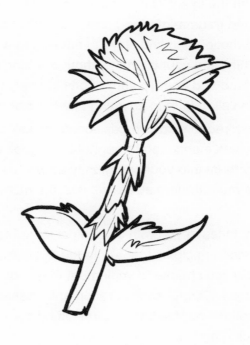

Chapter 20
Final Thoughts

A multitude of ideas in this manuscript have been presented with the intent of helping you begin to shape your thinking around trauma-informed care. Now it is up to you to take this information and find ways to adjust it to work best for you, your family, and your clients. Although writing this book took a lot of time and energy, your efforts to implement these ideas is more valuable than anything I have done in this text.

Be inspired toward compassionate action. Dive deeper into the therapies mentioned throughout this book and find ways to carry them into your community as well as your private practice. The more trauma aware we are, the more healing we can create.

I want to leave you with some final thoughts around the trauma-informed principles that are found throughout this book. No matter how you choose to implement these, do so with love and mindfulness. Careful consideration and intentional practice are the ingredients necessary to start shifting our society into a space of healing and community support.

Safety

We must work with our clients to help them feel safe. Certain herbs can help to support a healthy nervous system response. People can learn different plant medicines to use based on how they are feeling. Other modalities can be implemented to help our clients more frequently obtain a state of ventral vagal safety.

Plant medicine can be implemented to help support a healthy nervous system response. Certain herbs can help a person return to a ventral vagal state when they are struggling. I encourage my clients to become more aware of how the herbs interact with their emotions so they can begin independently choosing what to use based on how they feel.

Similarly, essential oils and flower essences can be used to encourage the body to return to a sense of safety. The need for different oils and flower essences can change with time, so learning to notice when a switch could be helpful will make your work more effective.

Finding ways to adjust movement therapy to feel safe can help a person to enjoy the benefits without feeling activated. Adjusting meditations to allow a person to get glimpses of the meditative state without dissociating is powerful. Changing Reiki and energy work practices to match the needs of your clients can help them feel more relaxed during the sessions.

Without safety, no healing can be done. Finding a place of safety usually takes consistent monitoring. Humans are not static and their needs may change. As a trauma-informed herbalist, you recognize this and work to meet people where they are. When you embrace this, you are well on your way to making a significant difference for your clients.

Choice

When implemented correctly, choice can be a powerful tool to help a person heal and regain confidence. Of course, sometimes choices can be overwhelming, so you must pay attention to what works best for each client. Accepting when a client tells you "no" allows them to retain their autonomy.

Bringing attention to a positive choice a client has made can reinforce the idea that they make good decisions.

Plant medicine provides several opportunities for choice to be implemented. There can be times when there are two herbs that could both work equally well for a client and they can choose. Choices with flower essences can be similar. In trauma-informed aromatherapy, choosing is key to the oil's success.

Helping clients build a toolbox of different lifestyle changes and other natural therapies can help them have appropriate options to choose from to keep their wellness. These little moments of freedom to choose may feel trivial, but it can help a client foster a feeling of autonomy and control over their health. These emotions can help a person continue to stay on a path of healing.

Choosing is something we take for granted until the choices are taken away. Many people who have been in abusive situations or other forms of traumatic experiences can feel they no longer are able to make choices. When appropriate, offering choice and support helps people to begin to regain a sense of autonomy and confidence

Collaboration

Holistic health services have always valued collaboration. Instead of talking at our clients, most of us have discussions with them. We can enhance our work by understanding what has worked for them, where their interests lie, and how they find our services in relation to their needs.

Discussing the actions of herbs, essential oils, and flower essences can help clients to see how the plant will benefit them the most. Getting feedback on how clients are feeling after starting different therapies can help us plan the next steps of their journey. Collaboration allows us to make sure that the recommendations are helping our clients efficiently hit their goals.

Working with clients to determine what other therapies would be helpful is a form of collaboration. Having regular ways to solicit feedback will allow you to improve the offerings you choose. Listen intently, and without ego, in order to be as supportive as possible.

When you actively pay attention to someone's preferences and allow them to have a voice in their care, you begin to develop a bond of trust. Maintaining that trust through transparency is vital. Clients who are able to trust you will be able to focus on their healing instead of worrying about your intentions.

Trustworthiness

Communication and transparency help to reduce concerns that you will take advantage of your clients. Being professional, maintaining a safe space, and enforcing appropriate boundaries are ways that you can practice trustworthiness with your clients. Consistently offering clear recommendations and expectations can help them feel confident you have their best interest at heart.

Communicate the purpose of each recommendation you offer to your clients. Depending on the client, you may go more or less in depth into the explanation. Some people want to know all the whys and hows while others just want to know that it is likely to help. Setting expectations of what the therapy can do will help clients feel confident that your recommendations are appropriate.

Being open with clients when you feel they need support from another professional can make a difference in how trustworthy you appear. It is a sign of strength when you are willing to send them to the practitioner that can help them the best. When this is done from a place of integrity, it builds a stronger healer-client relationship.

Remember, people will notice if you are not being genuine in your attempts to build trust. None of this work can be done from a place of deception and still produce long-term success. You must take an inventory of your intentions and do the inner work to make sure you are selflessly approaching this.

Empowerment

Recognizing your clients' strengths and helping them find accommodations that make natural therapies more accessible is the epitome of empowerment. Suggesting helpful changes and responding positively when clients ask for support is important for this process. Collaboration and choice go hand in hand with empowerment and these three principles should guide you when you are in the midst of a session.

Educating clients during sessions about different herbs and other therapies can help them to feel more in control of their healing journey. When they know more about what is helping them and why, it becomes easier for clients to independently find complementary practices that make healing more efficient. Many sessions I spend more time educating than I do outright recommending things for my clients.

Verbalizing different adjustments that clients can make during certain therapies can help empower them to change things when they become uncomfortable. It can also reinforce the positive results of a choice they have made. Pointing out the successes a person has, instead of focusing on all the ways they feel they have failed, helps to reinforce a sense of success on the healing journey.

Empowerment is a key aspect of clients becoming more confident in their healing. We can learn all sorts of different therapies and uses for herbs, but if we aren't helping clients feel they have some control over their wellness, our work falls flat. See how you can implement the things you've learned in this book to empower people around you to find healing.

Recognizing the needs of marginalized communities

Systemic discrimination issues change the effectiveness of our natural therapies. We cannot be successful trauma-informed herbalists if we cannot see this. Take time to read a couple of the books I recommended in the last chapter and see how you could do better.

Challenge your implicit bias. Follow professionals in marginalized communities who are working to shift the narrative. Take the Harvard tests I mentioned early on in the book.

Recognize there is a problem, but also take the time to figure out how to make things more equitable. Find ways to proactively accommodate others. Offer financially sensitive services and products. Amplify healers that are part of these communities. It's not going to fix everything, but If everyone did a little bit, the results would add up fast.

Now it's your turn

If we were to sum this book up in one phrase, it would be: choose mindful and compassionate action. We've discussed a lot of useful forms of plant medicine and other natural therapies. You now can see how many of these things can be adjusted to be trauma-informed. Commit to the paradigm shift and begin to make a difference in your community.

As you continue on your path, take what you've learned here and find ways to apply it to the situations you face at work and in your private life. Work to heal our communities through herbal medicine. Choose to be in the arena together with the rest of us who are offering trauma-informed support.

I wish you the best on this quest. Some days this work can feel overwhelming, so just remember those feelings are temporary. If you continue studying and growing as a trauma-informed herbalist, you will be contributing to deep healing that can resonate for generations to come.

Appendix
Recommended Reading List

In chapter nineteen, I recommended many books that can be helpful in understanding systematic discrimination and the struggles of many disenfranchised groups. That list starts on page 307. This recommended reading list is focused on trauma related books that can help you to further study the effects of trauma.

For those of you who are still struggling with trauma and activation, there are stories in several of these books that are difficult to read. I am not saying don't read them, but I am saying that it can be helpful to be aware and stop if you begin to feel activated. I had to put down most of these titles more than once, walk away, and return to the work later when I felt more centered.

The Body Keeps the Score

Dr. Bessel Van der Kolk's book. This is the popular title that has a lot of people paying closer attention to trauma and how it manifests. The body's role in the manifestation of trauma wasn't widely recognized until Dr. Van der Kolk wrote this masterpiece.

In an Unspoken Voice

Dr. Peter Levine's follow up to his original book, Waking the Tiger. The first couple of chapters are similar, but I feel this book goes into greater practical application of his ideas. Dr. Levine's work in somatic experiencing is groundbreaking, and this book feels like his magnum opus.

Polyvagal Safety

This is Dr. Stephen Porges' most recent book on polyvagal theory. It's a fantastic read that helps to discuss the idea that the perception of safety is paramount for healing. Pair this with Deb Dana's "Polyvagal Exercises for Safety and Connection" and you have a fantastic personal support plan.

Trauma Sensitive Mindfulness

For a more thorough discussion on trauma sensitive mindfulness, please consider reading the book "Trauma-Sensitive Mindfulness" by David Treleaven. His expertise on the topic is irreplaceable. He presents discussions around how to approach mindfulness, recognizing how trauma-informed care and equity for marginalized groups go hand in hand, and accepting the limitations of meditation.

Atlas of the Heart

Not trauma related, exactly, but this book helps us to expand our vocabulary around how we discuss emotions. Brené Brown does amazing emotions based research, and I believe this book can help us parse through our feelings and more clearly communicate with each other. The book leads to stronger connections, which are important to bring us to a place of ventral vagal safety.

About the Author

Elizabeth Guthrie, MPH, RYT 500 is a board certified wellness practitioner, clinical herbalist, and teacher in Birmingham, Alabama.

She holds a Bachelor's of Science in Complementary Medicine and has participated in creating research and leading activities at UAB hospital's integrative clinic.

Elizabeth's personal experiences led her to begin studying trauma and its effects on the body and mind.

Now she helps others to learn how natural wellness can be safely implemented as part of a trauma recovery journey.